MAN'S WORLD *digest*

No.2, being a digest of MAN'S WORLD Issue 9 / Jan 2023

Cover image: Skinless Frank (@skinless_frank on Instagram)

MAN'S WORLD
digest #2

CONTENTS

6 JESTER'S PRIVILEGE (AND THE FOOL WHO WILL SAVE THE UNIVERSE!)
Provocation by B.G. KUMBI

10 WHAT TODAY'S RIGHT GETS WRONG ABOUT MASCULINITY
Counterblast essay by JOHN MAC GHLIONN

16 MASCARA
Fiction by ALDIA

24 IT'S BIOLENINISM, STUPID
Essay by RAW EGG NATIONALIST

30 and 56 LET'S NOT DECLARE A PANDEMIC AMNESTY
Art and reflections by GIO PENNACCHIETTI

32 TRADITION AND THE INDIVIDUAL TALENT
Classic essay by T.S. ELIOT

40 SLAVES AND FREE MEN
Essay by SCOTT LOCKLIN

44 A STRANGE BEAUTY
Art by ALEXANDER ADAMS

48 LETTER FROM A FATHER TO HIS SON
Translation of a text by HENRY DE MONTHERLANT

60 THE RADICAL ARISTOCRAT OF HOLLYWOOD
Film with YAMNAYANAGE

MAN'S WORLD

RAW EGG NATIONALIST

editor-in-chief

RAW EGG NATIONALIST

editorial director

RAW EGG NATIONALIST

deputy editor

RAW EGG NATIONALIST

art director

RAW EGG NATIONALIST

deputy editor's assistant

RAW EGG NATIONALIST   *editor at large*

EDITORIAL

COPY: RAW EGG NATIONALIST

RESEARCH: RAW EGG NATIONALIST

STAFF: RAW EGG NATIONALIST

ART

RAW EGG NATIONALIST

senior art director

RAW EGG NATIONALIST

art coordinator

PUBLIC RELATIONS

RAW EGG NATIONALIST

vice president / director

ADVERTISING

GLOBAL: RAW EGG NATIONALIST

RAW EGG NATIONALIST *Your editor*
"Time for seconds!"

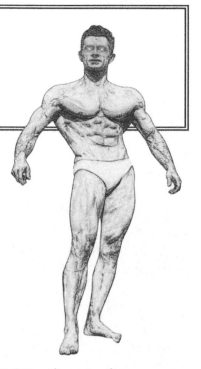

It's that time again, isn't it? "What time?" you ask. Time, I reply, for the return of the finest man's magazine in the world today. And what's more, that means it's time for another edition of the MAN'S WORLD Digest.

So welcome, my dear friends, to the second edition of the MAN'S WORLD Digest, being a handy little curated selection – curated by yours truly – of some of the best material from Issue Nine of MAN'S WORLD proper. Nine issues, a second Annual (available now from Antelope Hill!), a second Digest and the beginning of a third year. Wow!

What's in store for you then? First up to bat is B.G. KUMBI, otherwise known as the "philosopher of comedy". In a provocative provocation, he argues that laughter is truly the best medicine – and who are we to disagree? Then we have MAN'S WORLD's third Counterblast polemical essay, this time from my good friend JOHN MAC GHLIONN (who wrote a very nice profile of me for the Federalist recently). The Big Mac tells us exactly what the right gets wrong about masculinity, apropos of Senator Josh Hawley's new book. There's tremendous original fiction from ALDIA ("Mascara"), which is followed by an essay by your humble editor (yes, me!) on bioleninism. Bioleninism is the theory, first put forward by NRX OG Spandrell that the modern political game works by building a coalition of freaks and weirdos. Sounds plausible, doesn't it? Well, it is, and we need to find a way to change the rules of the game if we aren't to end up in the lesbian Bergen-Belsens prophesied by Bronze Age Pervert. Then what? This being MAN'S WORLD, we couldn't get by without some high-quality art, and thankfully we have GIO PENNACCHIETTI to provide it, with a visual essay in response to the *Atlantic*'s shameless call for a "pandemic amnesty". There's a reprint of T.S. Eliot's classic essay, "Tradition and the Individual Talent". SCOTT LOCKLIN goes back to the sources, to the ancient Greeks, to tell us the essential difference between free men and slaves. There's another great art essay from ALEXANDER ADAMS. Our penultimate piece is a translation of Henry De Montherlant's "Letter from a Father to His Son", in which he counsels his son — or any son — on how to be a man. Last, but by no means least, we have YAMNAYANAGE with a wonderful profile of filmmaker John Milius.

I hope you're hungry: it's time for seconds!

RAW EGG NATIONALIST (@babygravy9)

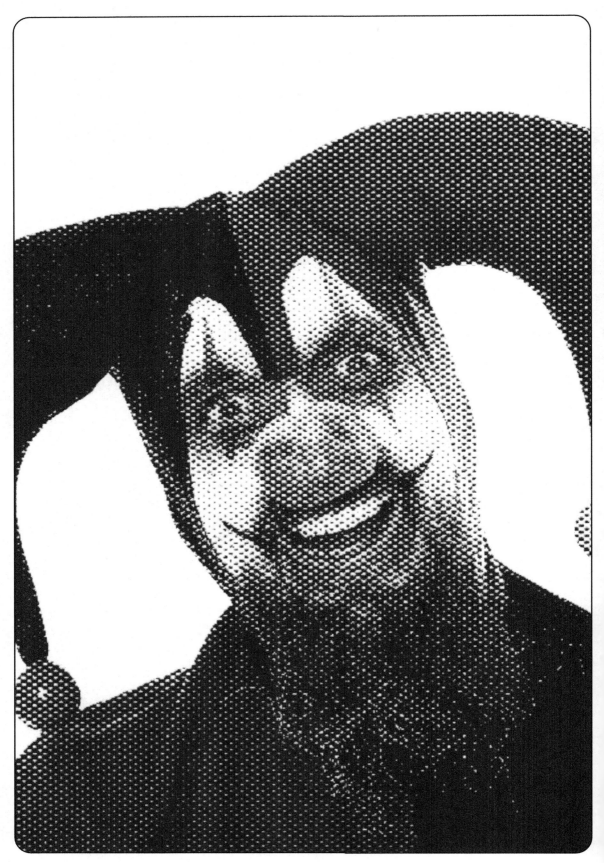

JESTER'S PRIVILEGE (AND THE FOOL WHO WILL SAVE THE UNIVERSE!)

provocation **BY B.G. KUMBI**

"Ridicule is man's most potent weapon" – Saul Alinsky, *Saul Alinsky's Rules for Radicals*

A truth, from the mouth of the devil himself. No, Saul Alinsky was no devil. I wouldn't give him such regard. Maybe a bubble of phlegm from the devil sneezing, briefly foaming to the surface, but bringing with it just a taste of *dark truth*. Truth in itself isn't necessarily good. The truth simply is. And there are two works of non-fiction literature that have told the truth about our reality better than any other: *Saul Alinsky's Rules for Radicals,* and Sun Tzu's *The Art of War*.

For whatever reason, we've found ourselves as beings in some place playing a great game that most don't, and never will, understand. The big questions have already been answered. If you're going looking for answers beyond those answers... well, I'll get to that, too. Entropy and natural selection are the rulers of this place. The game is simple: Become God before all the clocks melt.

It begins: The dice are cast: The single-celled organism forms in an ashen puddle and then another, and another, and the biggest one eats first, and eats all, until he is strong, stronger, *strongest*! Until he crawls from the slime: a beast with some chutzpah at last, no longer aimlessly colliding in dark waters, but equipped with limbs and claws and teeth to tear at new snacks. And out there, all across this great Earth, others have been coming out to play the game too. Some with wings to fly, some with fins to swim; some great feathered lizard gods, stomping about, unhinging their jaws to break the body and suck the candy goo from all that ever was. Imagine. Born to be a snack! What a brutal, twisted game we've found ourselves in, no?

The Earth, she goes around the sun, again and again, through collisions and explosions and great sheets of ice that seem never-ending, "A screaming comes across the sky" "Look!" down falls a glowing black balloon. Little gray men watch from far off stars through big binoculars. It's impossible! It's insurmountable! *This game... this game...* all creatures grit their teeth in some secret, withheld frustration, *is so unfair*.

Oh, it gets worse, so much worse. *Humans*. Swords and guns. Heads on pikes. Tongues ripped out. Torture. Fingernails pulled off. Such a high ceiling of suffering! War! War! War! May the most evil, most willing to gamble, take home all the spoils.

The Earth, she goes around the sun.

How much it all bleeds. Then goes to sleep. Sleep now. Close your eyes. Let the light fade from the Pleroma. And one day, the whole universe would seemingly shut off all her lights forever. But that wandering eye still peers through the windows, looking for anything left in the darkness.

That God, who only ever *looks*. It's all too delicate to touch. Too motherly an act to cradle in His arms and care for. So from an endless attic, through endless windows, he only ever peers: true neutral...

Quantum mechanics.

That's what He came up with to govern a game so absurd. Absurdity breeds absurdity and on and on. Or is He in that attic yet at all? Is it empty? Are those whispers and creaking floorboards only the wind? Are the molecules and pieces bouncing... *wait!*

Somewhere in the dark, there's a brief, stifled laugh. Is someone out there? And is he finding all of this horror... *funny!?*

Then it clearly hasn't all disappeared, just because the lights have gone out. No, there is a man standing at the edge of a great cliff over a stormy sea–– nothing but rocks and violent waves below him to trip down into the pitch dark if he dares take a step. And yet he laughs. *What am I!? Where and why have I found myself!? Why am I so afraid to die, yet can only smile and laugh!?* He already knows:

Because I am going to turn the lights on.

The Earth, she goes around the sun. The man he thinks, he schemes, he laughs. Nothing much seems to happen in this dark world. Every once in a while he finds himself in such a fit of joy and laughter, because as the millennia pass, he still knows it, in his heart, that still beats with that old bray: I am, I am, I– *phhht HAHAHAHA! How absurd!*

One day, one not so special day, still standing in the dark: it strikes him. Like a snap of the fingers. All so suddenly. He laughs more and more now. *How simple! How elegant! No one's out there! I'm no hero, I'm no God-- I'm simply a fool.* And so he finally devises a plan. *The* plan. A sort of plan only a fool would be silly enough to think would work. *Why, it's so simple. If the world is so dark and so dismal. I will just... I'll be the sunrise.*

A voice as sweet and as soft as rain speaks to him now through all that once was only hopelessness. "What a beautiful man you are... *Glockenschtork.*"

Yes! That's right! I have a name! Glockenschtork. A silly name for a silly man for a silly universe!

She breathes through his skin like a breezy wildfire. The light of the Pleroma comes shining through him. The universe is full of light. The sunrise has come. And not just one sunrise! So many! So many sunrises! Glockenschtork finally takes a step, and looks over the great cliffs that once surrounded him. But he is no longer The Fool. He has become something else. One of the *lost cards.* One of the purposefully buried cards. He has become *The Boundless Man.*

"Isn't it funny, Glockenschtork?" Sophia asks.

"Yes, of course. It's always *been* funny."

"There are many games, and many universes. There is goodness and cruelty. Hatred and love. And just a dash of some magic even a God can't touch with empires and armies and swords alone."

"It was a game of imagination," The Boundless Man states matter-of-factly.

"Why, yes, of course," Sophia says.

"They shouldn't have chosen someone with endless optimism to play it."

"Fate, Glockenschtork, is like a barbed wire, that drags us bleeding and screaming to where we need to go. Whether you can withstand the pain and hold on until the end is what determines whether you shall ever meet your most beautiful end. It is not guaranteed. You may have severed yourself from the string of fate any time you wished, had it become too much for you to bear. But you laughed instead. Every time. It wasn't guaranteed. You chose your courage.

In fact, most don't crack a smile."

"And what happens?" The Boundless Man asks. "If you let go?"

"Why, isn't that obvious? It's physical science."

Glockenschtorks laughs loudly. "I'm not very smart! I still don't know!"

Sophia smiles at him.

"What happens if you let *go*?"

Glockenschtork, still smiling, nods, eagerly, wanting to know.

"You fall forever."

He bursts out with such a laugh the whole universe seems to shake.

***

Here we find ourselves back as humans on Earth. Lowly, monkey creatures, afraid, cooped in our little hovels, hoarding our candies and gold. Pay a hundred dollars to write a message on a missile to fire into the face of another man! Another city burns. Another man of prominence is reduced to ashes with ridicule alone, stomped, stamped out by man's most potent weapon, and blown away like dust; and how deliberate, how intricately it was planned! Irony and snark and petty little quips. They wear down even giants as they turn joy into perversion. As we wait, and we wait, for some kind of miracle, or hero, to save us from all this fire…

Rejoice, I tell you!

For he has returned. He's not a billionaire, or anyone famous. But one day he did appear, called himself Glockenschtork, and said those same words that The Fool once spoke: *I'll be the sunrise.*

And now this game has been twisted once again. Who will become the greatest killing machine? Or who will sprout the prettiest orchid? A silly game of imagination! Not war. War will lose to imagination every time. War will lose to silliness, just as orchids grow through concrete and brick and glass. Not weaponized mockery. But laughter from that good place that blooms all outside of the attic like infinite fireworks, where we may fly and burst and turn to mist like the grass after a great rainstorm has worn down to a puddle! Boundless! To shimmer in the sunrise, like corral, mermaid fins, and dragon scales. Life once again has become a fairy tale. And to smile, so, so widely it almost hurts.

To feel so happy someday isn't impossible you know. To laugh in the dark may seem foolish at times – *Metanoia* they call it. Time is one great statue of a clown. Whether it be entropy or natural selection. Empires and despots: their hearts still beating somewhere in the sea. All their palaces shrunk to grains of sand.

Rejoice, I tell you. For *laughter* is man's most potent weapon. And there are some men who are simply too silly to sweep away like dust. He'll just make funny shapes as he flies through the air. And soon it's the one blowing so hard who finds himself angry and out of breath and on his knees. And there in the dust, in the air, unfettered by the weapons of war or words, he makes the shape of an orchid. Then a juggler, a jester, a clown, a glowing black balloon – a whole circus of lights!

One fool who can never be stamped out, or swept away by anyone. With a gesture, he sweeps the heavenly pavement himself.

Metanoia, they call it. Or was it *panache*? The Earth, she goes around.

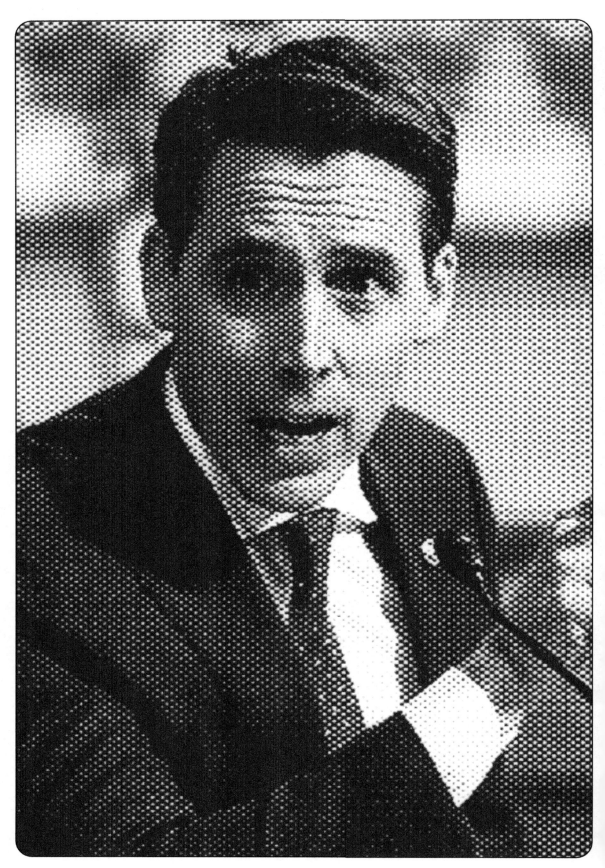

WHAT TODAY'S RIGHT GETS WRONG ABOUT MASCULINITY

essay **BY JOHN MAC GHLIONN**

The right is barking up the wrong tree when it comes to the problems belabouring today's men, says JOHN MAC GHLIONN

Henry David Thoreau famously said that "the mass of men lead lives of quiet desperation". A century and a half later, his words still resonate. In the US, men die by suicide 3.6 times more often than women. From Los Angeles to Louisiana, millions of American men are lonely and desperate. For years, masculinity, the set of attributes and behaviors that separate males from females, has been demonized. The vast majority of the demonization has come from left-leaning commentators, many of whom consider masculinity to be toxic. Instead of offering solutions to help the men of America, the Left offers nothing but ridicule and scorn. But what about those on the Right? What are they offering? More importantly, is what they're offering any good?

In short, no. Here's why.

Josh Hawley, the junior United States senator from Missouri, thinks he has a solution to the masculinity crisis sweeping across the land. The 42-year-old has a new book coming out soon, provocatively titled "Manhood: The Masculine Virtues Americans Need." According to the book's description on Amazon, the country's founders "believed that a republic depends on certain masculine virtues." Senator Hawley "calls on American men to stand up and embrace their God-given responsibility as husbands, fathers, and citizens," because a "free society that despises manhood will not remain free." Strong words. But, I ask, is Hawley qualified to offer prescriptions on masculinity?

This has nothing to do with him running away from a mob. Let's be honest, only idiots run towards a mob. Sadly, Hawley's philosophies ring hollow, largely because he is spouting 20th century ideas in a 21st century world. He is preaching a gospel of masculinity delivered through the prism of Christian nationalism. Hawley's advice comes at the very same time more and more Americans are turning away from all religions, Christianity included.

Hawley, like so many others on the right, speaks about the importance of marriage. Although the institution of marriage is very much the backbone of modern-day society, that backbone is badly damaged, a fact that seems to be lost on so many right-leaning commentators.

This is not the America your parents knew. No, this is post-marriage America. Not long from now, the unmarried will be the majority. As Aaron Clarey, the author of The Menu: Life Without the Opposite

Sex, says, post-marriage America will see people date "in perpetuity" until the day they die. Women, not men, are the reason why.

Unless you happen to live under a rock, you're probably familiar with the term "strong, independent woman." In the US, "strong independent women" rule with an iron fist. But what are these women independent of, exactly? In one word: men. As Mr. Clarey told me, on women's list of priorities, marriage now sits in 5th place. Their number one priority? Independence, basically a synonym for career.

This goes a long way to explaining why the country's marriage rate is at a 120-year low. Marriage has been demonized, and this demonization has a lot to with demonization of masculinity and men in general. Often referred to as a tool of the patriarchy, marriage, we're told, is an "inherently unfeminist institution," a construct that must be destroyed. Feminism, in its original form, may have helped women initially, but the metastasized version has destroyed many aspects of society. The idea of tearing men down to lift women up is, at best, silly. At worst, it's downright dangerous. Men and women are complimentary; we are better together than we are apart. An obvious point, for sure, but a point that is lost on so many American women.

I reached out to Rollo Tomassi, the best-selling author who has written extensively on the likes of intersexual dynamics and the institution of marriage, for comment on the matter. In The Rational Male – Religion, Tomassi refers to monogamous marriage as "one of the bedrocks of success for Western civilization." Marriage, he argues, was once "a good idea," but not anymore. Today, he told me, marriage is "one of the worst prospects imaginable for men," largely because society has moved from the idea of covenant marriages to contractual marriages. This is a point of vital importance that is rarely discussed.

Covenant marriages, in Tomassi's words, describe "how it should be done – religiously, personally, and devotionally." For millennia, covenant marriages were the rule. Today, however, contractual marriages are the norm. According to Tomassi, they are "the worst legal contractual liability a man can enter into." This is because the contractual marriage "is based on mutual support and an assurance that this support will continue even if the marriage itself dissolves."

Contractual marriages are closely associated with no-fault divorces. In simple terms, no-fault divorces don't require a showing of wrongdoing by either party. In 1970, Ronald Reagan, a notorious bed hopper, signed the no-fault divorce law into effect.

> **Today, American women find 80% of men physically unattractive. This is somewhat understandable. After all, 54 million men are overweight**

UNREALISTIC EXPECTATIONS

Today, American women find 80% of men physically unattractive. This is somewhat understandable. After all, 54 million men are overweight (34 million are obese). However, it must be noted that American women are not exactly the picture of health, with one in five now classified as obese. Less than a decade from now, one in two American adults will be obese. The United States is fast becoming a more objectively ugly country, and this ugliness will hurt men more than women.

You see, women are, by default, hypergamous. That is, they are more likely to want to marry into a higher caste or social group. In other words, men are more likely to settle for average or below average women. So, then, what does an above-average man look like in the eyes of an average or below average, American woman? Besides being physically attractive, a man must also be economically attractive. Perhaps you are familiar with the 666 rule, where a guy must be six foot tall, make six figures per year, and possess six pack abs. This is what women want. Now, ask yourself, how many American men do you know who tick all three boxes? How many tick one of these boxes? Not many, I imagine.

For the fortunate (or unfortunate) few that do pass the test and get married, I have even more bad news for you. Some seventy percent of divorces are now initiated by women (thanks, Ron). That number jumps to 90% among college-educated women. In modern-day America, women make up 60% of college students. Not only is it getting harder for men to find a respectable woman to marry, those who do find a wife are faced with a high chance of being divorced.

In *Modern Romance,* a book co-authored by the comedian Aziz Ansari and the sociologist Eric Klinenberg, the duo discuss the fact that marriage, not that long ago, was "an economic institution in which you were given a partnership for life in terms of children and social status and succession and companionship." Of course, modern day women "still want their partners to give them all these things, but in addition," wrote the authors, "they want men to be their best friend and their trusted confidant and their passionate lover to boot." Idealistic, delusional, call it what you will; expecting this from any person, be they male or female, is both selfish and unfair. This is a time when perfectionism is on the rise. One needn't be a psychologist to recognize the fact that the refusal to accept anything short of perfection is detrimental to society and romantic relationships.

Perfection is an illusion, but try telling this to millions of modern day women. While you're at it, try telling this to many on the right who do nothing but tell men to "man up", get married, and start a family.

> **Not only is it getting harder for men to find a respectable woman to marry, those who do find a wife are faced with a high chance of being divorced**

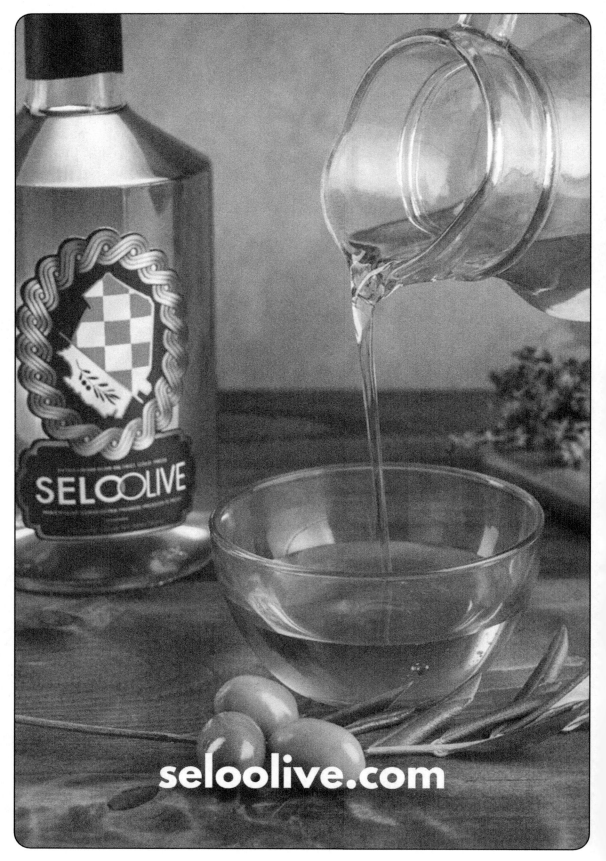

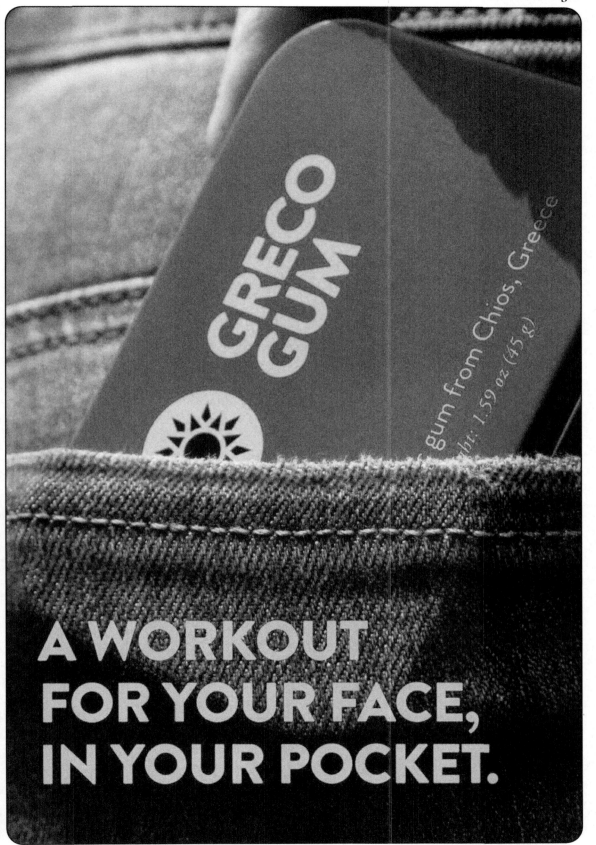

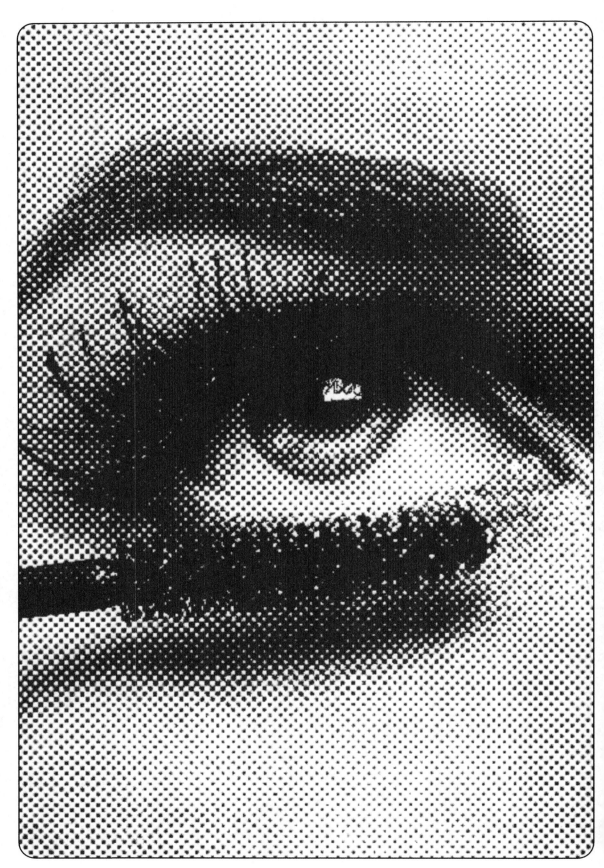

MASCARA

fiction **BY ALDIA**

In this exclusive short story for MAN'S WORLD, ALDIA (@aldiaskeep) introduces us to Mackey, a man who refuses to do himself any favours when it comes to the opposite sex

My friends say Mackey is utterly repulsive. He's blind in one eye and has the worst hairline I've ever seen, but he can bench 275 and has a great sense of humor. I see where they're coming from – I do – but all together, I don't think the man's too bad.

Last December, I'm busy with work and don't see much of anyone that month other than my girlfriend, Lys. On New Year's Day, my friend Fay throws a little get-together at her place, and I'm happy to see everyone again. My buddy Julian is there and a couple of Fay's coworkers too, as well as a garish creature I barely recognize as Mackey.

He's wearing blue mascara and earrings with little plastic devils; knee-high boots and designer jeans that look like dishrags; and a kimono shirt, printed with koi fish and Japanese characters. I ask Mackey what the Japanese get-up is for, and he gives me a knowing smile. I realize the shirt is a very old in-joke among our friends. The joke, I will add, is easy to explain but won't be funny to anyone but us. Lys and Julian think the shirt, and the joke, will be a good conversation starter. Fay even says to Mackey, "you look hot, you look good."

Mackey tells me a few girls have already commented on his mascara. I want to comment that none of those girls are dating him, and I want to tell him the shirt will *not* be funny when he explains it to his date. I want to tell him what Lys, Fay, and Julian *really* think of his looks—and I want to rip off all of Mackey's clothes.

Now that's a thought I never thought I'd have.

***

One day, Mackey drops a picture of himself in the group chat. He's cock-eyed and sticking his tongue out, wearing his kanji shirt and the pair of devil earrings.

on my way to another tinder date, he says below the photo. *wish me luck*

Then the supplicants come in their blubbering hordes.

ur gonna kill it. show of that big dick energy, Fay says.

you don't need any luck. you gots it, my girlfriend says.

Julian adds on too. *my mans, she'd be an idiot not to date you.*

Naturally, Mackey never sees that girl again, nor any girl this month. But in all these photos, he looks undeniably happy, so should I really be so upset?

***

A couple weeks later, everyone but me is at some dive bar next to Fay's place. I get a blurry selfie of my girlfriend and Mackey. He has his arms wrapped around her, his mascara's running down his face like a clown doused with a bucket of water. It's no surprise he's crying. This is what you get for dressing like that. I laugh, until white-hot pain shoots up from my knee to my spine.

I'm baffled. I've felt pity before, but I don't remember it being *excruciating*. Maybe this is real pity. Not self-pity or the media-enforced pity you feel hearing about a famine a thousand miles away. I'm a little disgusted with myself for having laughed, but I certainly got what I deserved. I just don't want to feel that again.

So I give Lys a call. She's in a noisy corner of the bar and says Mackey's drunk and been hugging her all night. I hear him moaning in the background, "I'm so lonely, I'm so lonely…"

The nerves in my leg and back are tingling. I go off on Lys. "Okay, give the man a hug or two, yes, definitely. But Christ alive, that guy needs to stop wearing mascara and get rid of that fucking shirt! I know that joke means a lot to him… but it's not funny. It's not funny anymore, you need to tell him that. You can't laugh when he brings it up either, not even a little bit. I swear to God, Mackey is a good guy, he's not bad looking either. He lifts too! This isn't rocket science, I'm no womanizer myself, but anyone can see what's wrong here. Tell Mackey to stop with this kimono bull-"

Lys interrupts me. She wants me to pick her up from the bar because Mackey's making her uncomfortable. I harangue Lys until she admits to being selfish and agrees to be there for Mackey, if only for one night. I tell her goodnight then hang up and go to bed, but the image of mascara running down Mackey's face keeps me up.

***

A week later, we're at another dive bar. It's the kind of place you go to when you want the scents and noises to fill your head and push the bad thoughts out. There's a pool table, which is great, because there aren't any women. This is Lys and Fay's favorite bar, because the drinks are cheap, and the gay men are harmless. Mackey's there too, in his Japanese shirt, along with Julian and a couple of Fay's coworkers. Fay, after one round of pool, goes outside to smoke and doesn't come back. My girlfriend ditches me to chat with Fay and her friend, so Mackey and I play some pool.

> **I've felt pity before, but I don't remember it being *excruciating*. Maybe this is real pity. Not self-pity or the media-enforced pity you feel hearing about a famine a thousand miles away**

"There's not many girls here, are they?" Mackey says after sinking another shot.

I laugh. "You don't say…"

"I'll tell you, man. It's not easy as people tell you."

I can tell the liquor has loosened him up, so I ask, "What isn't easy?"

I can see he debates telling me. "Would you judge me if I said it isn't like the movies?"

"No, never," I say.

"You're a bad liar." He chuckles and tells me anyways. "I really did think I'd meet someone when I went back to school, but man – those girls!" He puts the pool stick across his shoulders. "I'd rather they just ignore me. The nice ones, I mean. Cos' they make you believe there's something good about yourself, deep down, like there's something they see in you that no one else does. But every time… they just… they always keep you an arm's length away! I can't figure them out, man!"

I'd have thought if Mackey knew this, he'd be a little better off.

After sinking another ball, he goes on a little more. "Fay is always telling me how the guys she goes out with put up such an act to get in her pants."

"Does it work?" I ask.

"No," Mackey says.

"So she tells you."

Mackey grinds the chalk on the end of his stick. "What I'm trying to say is: you have to be yourself. You've got to be real."

"And you've got to go to a bar with a woman," I say as I line up another shot.

Of course, when I miss it, Mackey laughs. "You've got less balls in tonight than you've had girlfriends."

There's that great sense of humor.

I lose all three games.

***

Hanging over the patio is a fine gray mélange of cigarette smoke, marijuana, and Jul vapor. If there isn't already a subsection in the Chemical Weapons Convention regarding this substance, someone, please, put one in.

Mackey and I pass through the smog and sit down at the table with everyone else. Fay is handing a joint to my girlfriend, who nervously glances at me before declining and passing it to Julian. Fay's coworkers are already rolling another. They're thin, bag-eyed creatures, skin pocked from years of drug abuse. They're having a great time, telling us how they overdosed in the bathroom of a Tame Impala concert. In short, they are esteemed company.

Around one in the morning, this Mexican guy walks up to Mackey and says, "Hey, I love your mascara. I fuck with that so much." He's wearing a diaphanous pink scarf around his head, wrapped like a loose hijab. He doesn't quite have a lisp, but there's enough of one to tip me off.

His gay and Chicano accents clash.

"Oh, thanks, I did it in the car ten minutes before coming here," Mackey says. I can tell from the way he's talking, Mackey's wasted.

"Dude, it's good. Like, really good." The man in the scarf is stepping left and right, moving his hands up and down. Whatever he's on, it's strong, and I feel a deep, almost spiritual disharmony watching him gesticulate as he flirts with Mackey. "I like doing mine with the purple eyeliner sometimes, you know? It looks good at the club, you know?"

"I like your scarf!" my girlfriend says.

"Oh, thank you!" He does a pirouette. "I got it today at Goodwill…"

"Hey, man," I say to him. "Are you gay?"

My friends stop talking. Fay and Lys are mortified. Fay's coworkers and Julian are holding back laughter. Mackey looks somewhere in between, but I can't decipher his expression.

"Me?" The man in the scarf points a finger at himself. "No, ah, bro, I'm not into dudes…

Why? Are you?"

"Asking for my friend there," I say, surprised the man outright said no.

Maybe he's lying, maybe he *is* gay. I'm not so sure. I am, however, a hundred percent certain he'd suck a row of cocks for a baggie of PCP. Fay and her friends know it too. Fay's posture becomes withdrawn, turned away from the man in the scarf, trying to ignore him and trying harder to ignore what I said to him. She passes the joint to the friend of hers sitting furthest away from the outsider.

"I get it, I get it, it's cool, it's cool." The man in the scarf spins on the ball of his heel. "I fuck with gay people, though. I fuck with trans people too, you know? Trans rights, baby! If you don't believe in trans rights, get ready for these hands." He throws a few punches in the air above Mackey's head. "I fuck with trans people, I fuck with everybody…"

"Hey, man, what're you on?" I ask, trying not to laugh, "And what would you do for more of it?"

His eyes go wide. "I'm not on anything… for real, dude… I'm high on life, baby… you know what I mean?"

Fay and her friends start talking loudly. It's a very specific, personal conversation that completely embargos the man in scarf from joining. When he leaves, it's business as usual, and Fay's friends—who've been telling stories about their near-death drug experiences all night— look at me and smile with their rotten heroin teeth.

I do my best to smile back at them, though I am feeling very depressed. All these friends of mine, Julian, Lys, Mackey, Fay – who all have Pride bumper stickers and rainbow flags on the walls of their rooms – say nothing as I expel the man in the pink hijab from our conversation with a joke about his sexuality. This is because, my friends, when their little urbanite ecosystem is disturbed, they don't care what the disturbance is or how it's removed. All that matters is that it's gone.

And when I talk to Mackey about his looks, *I* will be the man in the scarf. I'll be a disturbance to his happy little thoughts, and he'll want me removed from his happy little ecosystem.

I excuse myself from the table and leave the bar, deciding it's just not worth it.

***

That night, I'm up late thinking what to do about Mackey, going back and forth with myself: tell him, don't tell him… arguments, counterpoints… actions and consequences… It's five in the morning when a warm feeling of clarity washes over me and realize: I have no right to tell Mackey what's good for him. I'm not sure I know how to live my own life, so what right do I have to tell Mackey how to live his? This just isn't my fight—it's Mackey's, to win or to lose. He's a grown man and can help himself. I don't feel much better about this revelation, but at the very least, I can get some sleep.

***

It's been a few months since I stopped going to bars with the gang. Today, however, is Fay's birthday, so I want to be there for the festivities. The bar we're at is cheap, dirty, and full of ugly people. Fay, Mackey, and Julian commiserate they haven't found a soulmate amidst the wretches and freaks. I agree with them: not even *they* deserve the twisted lumps of flesh we're surrounded by tonight.

My advice to them is a ménage à trois. They are not amused. I'm shoo-ed away, so they ask Lys for advice instead. I'm laughing under my breath because I know they've never taken anyone's advice and never will. They've never lowered their standards: they don't go to bars with people their age. Their sexualities change from month to month, but always go for 7's, 8's, and 9's. They go to dive bars with pool tables and karaoke machines because that's their happy little ecosystem and they don't want it disturbed.

When I go back to the table, Mackey's there, sitting by himself. He's staring into the eye of his whiskey glass, looking at the very end of his rope. His shirt is open to his navel, he's got the devils on his ears tonight.

And in the shadows of the bar, his mascara makes his eyes look like empty, black sockets.

I almost topple over. After all I did to eschew that feeling, here it is again. Surging up my leg, into my spine, and crashing into base of my skull. I get off my legs as quickly as I can, sitting at the barstool across from Mackey.

"Scene's kind of dead, isn't it?" I say making small talk.

"It's alright." There's a shot or two in him, but he's not that drunk.

"There're girls here, at least, but they're not really our age. Don't know if that matters to you. If you're just here to hang out with friends, it doesn't, but if you're trying to meet someone, well..."

"I'm trying to, yeah."

I see the tears forming. God, he really is trying.

Truly, the things men do for women are disgraceful, and the things women abet men in doing are even more despicable. I've long since accepted I can't do anything about either. The only thing I have control over is myself, but it seems tonight I don't have even that.

"To be honest, Mackey, I don't know if this is the right look for meeting girls," I say. "The mascara, the earrings, the kimono shirt—that joke, Mackey… It's been *three years*, it's just not funny anymore. I know it means a lot to you, but what will it mean to her? At best, nothing. At worst, a reason not to give you a chance. Let me put this in perspective: Fay can sleep with you. Or she can sleep with a thirty-two-year-old salaryman who has expendable income, a Porsche on lease, and a two-bedroom apartment that's on the other side of town from her parents' house. You don't have *any* of that, so you better look the part." I wipe the sweat off my forehead. "Fay doesn't know what she's talking about. You can be as superficial as you want, but—at the very least—if you don't look like someone she wants to fuck, there's nothing you have your competition doesn't."

Mackey sits there—gapes at me—like a sheep before slaughter. Cross-eyed, staring straight down the barrel of a bolt gun. He nods and bats his clumpy eyelashes, but I'm not sure he registers what I'm saying in the English language.

"Let's go to a bar that has girls our age, eh?" I slap him on the shoulder. "We'll dress up. Jeans and a nice dress shirt. Back to basics."

Mackey bobs his head with shiny, marble eyes. Something about his very peaceful expression makes me extremely nervous, so I start talking faster.

"I'm not to trying to hurt you, man. You've got a lot going for you: you work out, that's a leg up on most guys – and you're funny. I got way too lucky with Lys, we've been together four years now. If I wasn't with her, I'd be in the same boat as you. God knows I'd consider all the possibilities!"

I swallow and stare back at Mackey, badly wanting him to respond. I want him to say or do something other than nod and blink. Mackey, for God's sake, say something. Tell me I'm wrong! Tell me I'm right, start crying, start yelling… Do something, but don't sit there and look like a sheep!

"So, yeah," I say. "Let's go out some time… okay? You, me, and couple other of the boys. Got it?"

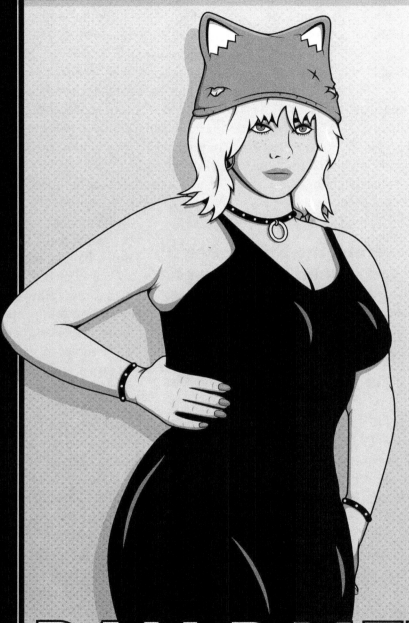

"Yeah, got it," he says.

I spend the rest of the night dodging conversations and thinking about what I said, but the more I play the conversation back, the more the words and sentences change. I'm tempted with all the different things I could've said and the hundred possibilities one word less or one word more could've amounted to. There's the possibility Mackey thanks me and burns the shirt. There's the possibility Mackey burst into tears then burns the shirt. Then, of course, there's the possibility Mackey spits in my face, breaks his whiskey glass on my head, then walks out of the bar and burns the shirt.

***

It's a few weeks before I see Mackey again. One night, when everyone else is busy, he insists we go to a bar downtown to talk. I listen to what he has to say, say something supportive, and then I walk up to a couple of girls and ask if they want to get a drink with my buddy and me. They say, "Why not?" and join us at the bar. One of the girls asks Mackey about his shirt, so he tells them story, the full story, and when it's over, they *burst into hysterics*. Everyone in the bar – the pretty girls to the toothless addicts – all the wretches and freak are laughing. Mackey laughs so hard he cries; I tell him his mascara's running, and when he goes to the bathroom to fix it, I make sure to sit down before I start laughing too.

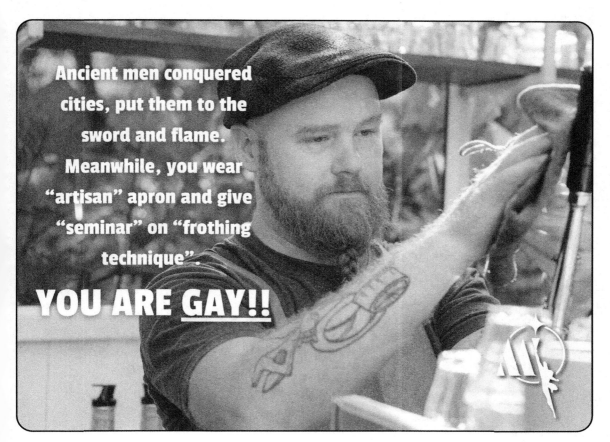

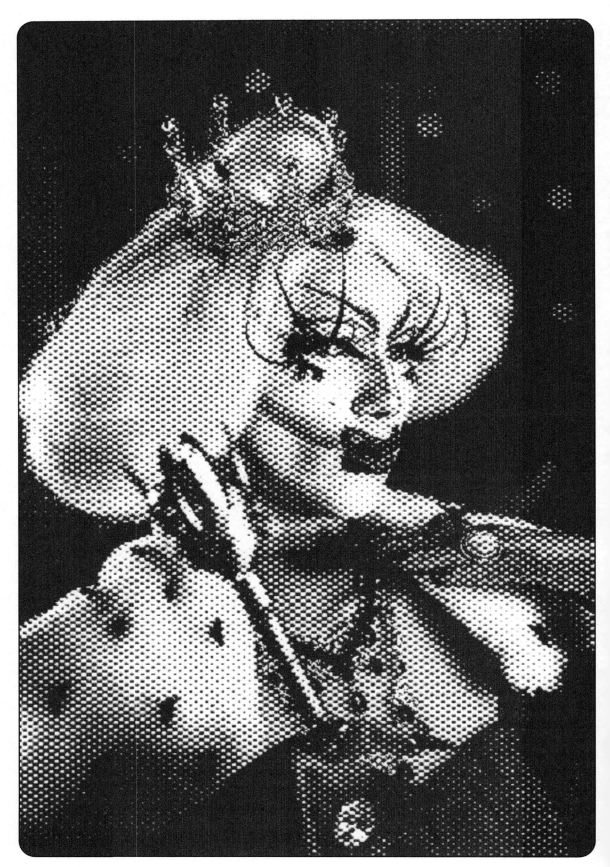

IT'S BIOLENINISM, STUPID

essay BY RAW EGG NATIONALIST

The rules of politics today are the rules of bioleninism, says RAW EGG NATIONALIST, and that's why things are only going to get worse

A spectre is haunting Europe – the spectre of bioleninism… Actually, bioleninism is haunting the entire Western world, not just Europe but also, and especially, the US. As each new day brings fresh rainbow-coloured bursts of insanity, so it also brings fresh confirmation that bioleninism is the main strategy our enemies, and even our supposed allies, are using to win at politics today.

Just what kind of things am I talking about? Here are a few examples.

The LGBTQ+ wing of the British Conservative party handing out badges with the slogan "Tories Cum" on them – a cunning play on the popular "Tory scum" jibe – at the party's annual conference. Yes, that's bioleninism. For sure.

What about the Somali takeover of the American Midwest, and the strange blend of progressivism and Third World tribalism we see embodied in figures like Ilhan Omar? Yes, that's bioleninism too. 100%.

Or what about the increasingly visible attempts to rebrand paedophiles as "minor-attracted persons" and, not only that, to represent their "rights" politically and even legalise their evil behaviour? You know what I'm going to say, don't you? (No, I wasn't going to say *that* – at least not out loud…). Yes: bioleninism again.

As disparate as these phenomena might seem at first glance, they all share an underlying logic, a political modus operandi, that unites them. Anon supremo Spandrell first laid bare those inner workings in three concise, but extremely incisive, posts on his blog in 2017, which were later packaged together as an ebook (available from archive.org, for instance). I can't recommend them enough.

The theory has stood the test of time and continues to provide a compelling explanation for why politics in the West, and especially the US, is now the way it is. By which I mean, why politics is a hideous demoralising shitshow if you're a half-competent man of European descent. More importantly, it explains why things are continuing, and will continue, to get worse.

Here's a question we'd all like to know the answer to: Why does the right keep losing, even when it wins elections? While the mainstream right will happily take each momentary success as a meaningful victory, seen in a broader span the general trend is so obviously down and away from anything that, say, Edmund Burke or a genuine traditionalist would recognise as worth defending or striving towards. The oft-made quip that in ten years' time conservatives will just be defending the shit progressives are pushing today, is all-too true: the progressive front line will be a conservative redoubt, a "principled" stand, by the end of the decade. And so nothing is preserved, nothing is protected, nothing conserved.

And why is that? It's quite simple: because bioleninism is the name of the game now. Bioleninism is the only way to guarantee political success – or at least it's widely acknowledged as the most effective way to do so. Which means we have "conservative" parties importing record numbers of foreign migrants, waving the rainbow flag at every opportunity and happily aiding and abetting the destruction of the past, one monument after another.

Like many, if not all, of the best theories of political behaviour, the bioleninism thesis is simple, but has explanatory power well beyond the sum of its parts. All it takes is a very basic model of behaviour at both the plebian and the elite level, informed by an historical account of Leninism's fortunes inside and outside the Soviet Union.

It's worth saying that, regardless of what you think of Lenin himself, Leninism has been one of the most fantastically successful political doctrines in modern history. It works, basically, because it appeals to the status-seeking module we all have in our brains, which motivates our behaviour to a greater or lesser extent. And Leninism works *so* well, because it promises status to a very particular demographic: those who have little or none.

These are precisely the people who will fight most ruthlessly to gain status, especially if it comes at the expense of hated groups ("the bourgeoisie", the aristocracy). By promising status in such a way, the revolutionary vanguard secures deep loyalty from a mass of low-status groups who would, in a very real sense, be lost without them.

Leninism consolidates political power, then, through the creation of a "coalition of the fringes" – a motley crew of the downtrodden, the dispossessed, and, of course, the deviant and the diseased. Modern societies generally produce such people in large numbers, and pre-Revolutionary Russia was certainly no exception. Note that such people are not simply "workers", as the romanticisers of the Revolution would have it. In fact, they're much more likely to be shirkers than workers. If you don't know or believe that quite literally some of the worst people in the world – and I don't mean Lenin, Trotsky, Dzerzhinsky or Stalin – were responsible for turning Russia red, I'd suggest you read Always with Honor, the memoir of White general Pyotr Wrangel, and learn how the prisons and the asylums were emptied by the communists to provide troops for the cause. And not just any troops, as I say, but warped, hateful fanatics who would do the dirty work of revolution with a twinkle in their eye and a spring in their step. Oswald Spengler (*The Hour of Decision*) also provides useful commentary on this "quality" of the real revolutionaries of 1917.

In the West, however, class war very

> **Regardless of what you think of Lenin himself, Leninism has been one of the most fantastically successful political doctrines in modern history**

quickly ceased to have any of the motive force it held in Tsarist Russia. The unheralded prosperity of the 1950s and 1960s forced the left to find a different basis upon which to promise increased status and thus consolidate power. Eventually, biology – the given natural facts that separate people regardless of prosperity – became that new basis. And what a basis! Thus followed the "liberation" of women; then gay "liberation" and "liberation" of ethnic minorities; and now, in 2022, the bioleninists are promising more of the same to pedophiles, practitioners of bestiality, grown men who choose to wear diapers, and Twitch streamers.

The bioleninism thesis works for another reason, too. It doesn't posit that we ended up with Leninism on steroids – perhaps "Leninism on puberty blockers and Zoloft" might be a better epithet – through some grand conspiracy. This wasn't all planned down to the last detail. Well, some parts of it were. Gramsci's Long March through the Institutions, by means of which the West's cultural and political institutions would be infiltrated and subverted from the inside, was definitely planned, and it's worked catastrophically well in giving progressives a near-impregnable series of bases from which to sally forth and piss, vomit and shit over everything in sight. But the pivot to a biological basis for Leninism was, nevertheless, a largely organic response to the failure of traditional Marxism to achieve revolution in the West in the manner Marx had predicted.

A large part of it is also just the nature of mass participatory democracy. As Spandrell says, the tendency of democracy is always to the left, precisely because the way to keep winning the democratic game is to appeal to ever-broader demo-

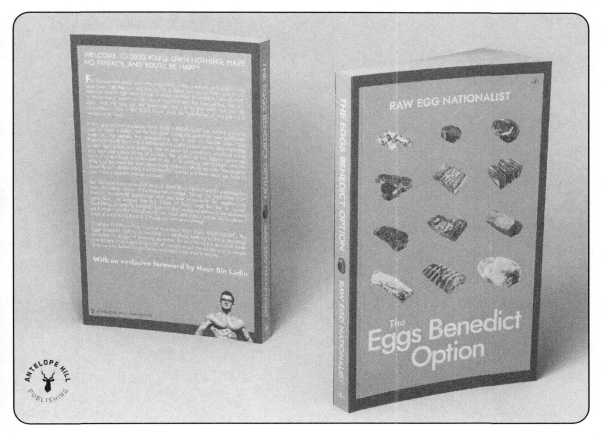

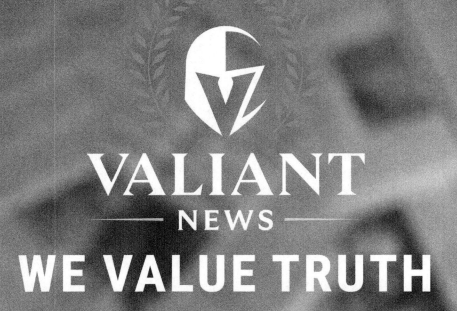

graphics. This fatal tendency of democratic rule was, of course, known to the ancients, and it's why prudent men of the past, including the American Founding Fathers, established all sorts of checks and balances against the rule of sheer quantity. It's no surprise, then, that the electoral college is now seen as an impediment to "real" democracy that must be done away with – since it really is an impediment and was always intended to be such.

If indeed there is a kind of Leninism baked into the system, this of course begs the question whether we must rid ourselves of the system if we want to be rid of biolenism once and for all. Spandrell doesn't shy away from this question or others about the future of politics in the West. But I'm not here just to explain the theory, I also want to expand it myself.

For one thing, it's clear that the physical and spiritual crisis of masculinity in the West – falling testosterone levels, rising infertility, depression and a general lack of purpose for men – is an essential prop of the bioleninist regime today.

Spandrell notes that, if bioleninism is anything, it's a revolt against male competency, and to the extent that the regime can actively discredit and demoralise young men, especially young men of European descent, it does. There can be no doubt that a powerful aid to this evil aim is the increasingly toxic environment we inhabit, which is feminising men in alarming ways and with alarming speed. This was one of the principal focuses of the Tucker Carlson documentary *The End of Men*, which was broadcast in October and which I and some of my Twitter friends featured in heavily.

We might even call this the regime's secret weapon, a kind of dirty war. Whether deliberately cultivated or not, this chemical warfare serves to reinforce, in the most-wide ranging manner, the regime's attempts to marginalise young men. And one thing that's abundantly clear from the reaction to the Tucker documentary – from the refusal of commentators to entertain the idea that certain chemicals have endocrine-disrupting effects, or that there's even a crisis of masculinity in the first place – is that actually this is something the regime is totally fine with. "The crisis of masculinity isn't happening, and here's why it's a good thing that it is."

Since the release of *The End of Men*, and my subsequent appearance on *Tonight with Tucker Carlson*, I've come in for criticism from certain segments of the online right for diverting attention towards "trivial" or "non-core" issues (i.e. health and fitness, aesthetics). Some of this is undoubtedly sour grapes; some of it, unfamiliarity with my work; and some, just plain ol' retardation (filter your water, people!). The truth, as I've tried to make explicit here, is that the health of young men is not a distraction from the real issues of our day. A mass movement focusing on health and fitness will not just make the right wing attractive again, which it has no excuse not to be and indeed must be if it is ever to succeed; such a movement will also strike at the heart of the bioleninist regime that is drawing the West deeper and deeper into the widening gyre.

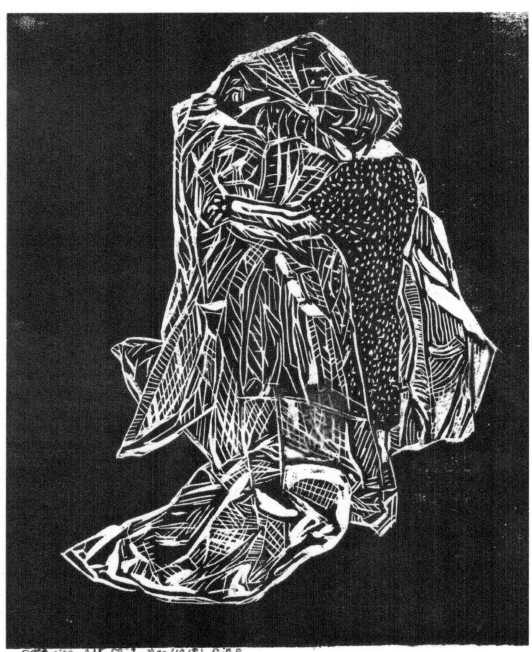

LET'S NOT DECLARE A PANDEMIC AMNESTY

art BY GIO PENNACCHIETTI

During the middle of lockdown I made a woodcut of a photo I saw floating around social media. It was of a woman hugging her elderly loved ones fully masked through a sheet of plastic. It reminded me of the post World War 1 woodcuts of German Expressionist Kathe Kollwitz. Women clutching on to men and children in solemn, fearful embrace, gaunt and ghostly shells of people yearning for warmth and comfort in the wake of mass tragedy. Death hanging in the air through the stark chiaroscuro of ink areas. It is but one small image, in the multitude of images I feel that I must depict as an artist. For this is the price of forgetting, one that that work of art does in remembrance of things past. Those covered and masked figures disappearing into a plastic sheet, a mass of feelings not truly felt, and human connection irretrievably interrupted. To forget is not an act of mass compassion and amnesty, but a betrayal of our humanity.

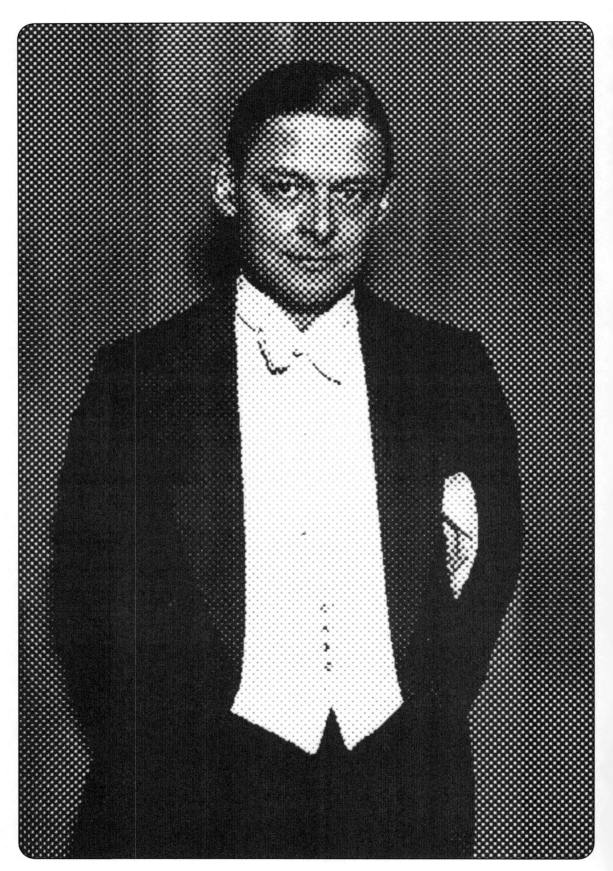

TRADITION AND THE INDIVIDUAL TALENT

classic essay **BY T.S. ELIOT**

Following on from last issue's inaugural *From the Archives* essay, we have T.S. Eliot's "Tradition and the Individual Talent." Arguably Eliot's most influential essay, "Tradition and the Individual Talent" is essential reading for all radical traditionalists who want to understand the relationship between the individual — especially but not exclusively the individual artist — and the broader tradition. The essay was first published in 1919, and soon after included in his collection of essays *The Sacred Wood: Essays on Poetry and Criticism* (1920). Perhaps the most important idea, for our purposes, that Eliot develops here is his notion that the past, i.e. tradition, is always actually present in the present. What we do in the present is or must be in reference to all that has come before; but at the same time, what we do retroactively alters tradition (even if only ever so slightly). Tradition, then, is not the dead weight of the past, but a living thing which changes with time.

In English writing we seldom speak of tradition, though we occasionally apply its name in deploring its absence. We cannot refer to "the tradition" or to "a tradition"; at most, we employ the adjective in saying that the poetry of So-and-so is "traditional" or even "too traditional." Seldom, perhaps, does the word appear except in a phrase of censure. If otherwise, it is vaguely approbative, with the implication, as to the work approved, of some pleasing archaeological reconstruction. You can hardly make the word agreeable to English ears without this comfortable reference to the reassuring science of archaeology.

Certainly the word is not likely to appear in our appreciations of living or dead writers. Every nation, every race, has not only its own creative, but its own critical turn of mind; and is even more oblivious of the shortcomings and limitations of its critical habits than of those of its creative genius. We know, or think we know, from the enormous mass of critical writing that has appeared in the French language the critical method or habit of the French; we only conclude (we are such unconscious people) that the French are "more critical" than we, and sometimes even plume ourselves a little with the fact, as if the French were the less spontaneous. Perhaps they are; but we might remind ourselves that criticism is as inevitable as breathing, and that we should be none the worse for articulating what passes in our minds when we read a book and feel an emotion about it, for criticizing our own minds in their work of criticism. One of the facts that might come to light in this process is our tendency to insist, when we praise a poet, upon those aspects of his work in which he least resembles any one else. In these aspects or parts of his work we pretend to find what is individual, what is the peculiar essence of the man. We dwell with satisfaction upon the poet's difference from his predecessors, especially his immediate predecessors; we endeavour to find something that can be isolated in order to be enjoyed. Whereas if we approach a poet without this prejudice we shall often find that not only the best, but the most individual parts of his work may be those in which the dead poets, his ancestors, assert their immortality most vigorously. And I do not mean the impressionable period of adolescence, but the period of full maturity.

Yet if the only form of tradition, of handing down, consisted in following the ways of the immediate generation before us in a blind or timid adherence to its successes, "tradition" should positively be discouraged. We have seen many such simple currents soon lost in the sand; and novelty is better than repetition. Tradition is a matter of much wider significance. It cannot be inherited, and if you want it you must obtain it by great labour. It involves, in the first place, the historical sense, which we may call nearly indispensable to any one who would continue to be a poet beyond his twenty-fifth year; and the historical sense involves a perception, not only of the pastness of the past, but of its presence; the historical sense compels a man to write not merely with his own generation in his bones, but with a feeling that the whole of the literature of Europe from Homer and within it the whole of the literature of his own country has a simultaneous existence and composes a simultaneous order. This historical sense, which is a sense of the timeless as well as of the temporal and of the timeless and of the temporal together, is what makes a writer traditional. And it is at the same time what makes a writer most acutely conscious of his place in time, of his own contemporaneity.

No poet, no artist of any art, has his complete meaning alone. His significance, his appreciation is the appreciation of his relation to the dead poets and artists. You cannot value him alone; you must set him, for contrast and comparison, among the dead. I mean this as a principle of aesthetic, not merely historical, criticism. The necessity that he shall conform, that he shall cohere, is not onesided; what happens when a new work of art is created is something that happens simultaneously to all the works of art which preceded it. The existing monuments form an ideal order among themselves, which is modified by the introduction of the new (the really new) work of art among them. The existing order is complete before the new work arrives; for order to persist after the supervention of novelty, the whole existing order must be, if ever so slightly, altered; and so the relations, proportions, values of each work of art toward the whole are readjusted; and this is conformity between the old and the new. Whoever has approved this idea of order, of the form of European, of English literature will not find it preposterous that the past should be altered by the present as much as the present is directed by the past. And the poet who is aware of this will be aware of great difficulties and responsibilities.

In a peculiar sense he will be aware also that he must inevitably be judged by the standards of the past. I say judged, not amputated, by them; not judged to be as

> **The whole of the literature of Europe from Homer and within it the whole of the literature of his own country has a simultaneous existence and composes a simultaneous order**

good as, or worse or better than, the dead; and certainly not judged by the canons of dead critics. It is a judgment, a comparison, in which two things are measured by each other. To conform merely would be for the new work not really to conform at all; it would not be new, and would therefore not be a work of art. And we do not quite say that the new is more valuable because it fits in; but its fitting in is a test of its value—a test, it is true, which can only be slowly and cautiously applied, for we are none of us infallible judges of conformity. We say: it appears to conform, and is perhaps individual, or it appears individual, and many conform; but we are hardly likely to find that it is one and not the other.

To proceed to a more intelligible exposition of the relation of the poet to the past: he can neither take the past as a lump, an indiscriminate bolus, nor can he form himself wholly on one or two private admirations, nor can he form himself wholly upon one preferred period. The first course is inadmissible, the second is an important experience of youth, and the third is a pleasant and highly desirable supplement. The poet must be very conscious of the main current, which does not at all flow invariably through the most distinguished reputations. He must be quite aware of the obvious fact that art never improves, but that the material of art is never quite the same. He must be aware that the mind of Europe—the mind of his own country—a mind which he learns in time to be much more important than his own private mind—is a mind which changes, and that this change is a development which abandons nothing en route, which does not superannuate either Shakespeare, or Homer, or the rock drawing of the Magdalenian draughtsmen. That this development, refinement perhaps, complication certainly, is not, from the point of view of the artist, any improvement. Perhaps not even an improvement from the point of view of the psychologist or not to the extent which we imagine; perhaps only in the end based upon a complication in economics and machinery. But the difference between the present and the past is that the conscious present is an awareness of the past in a way and to an extent which the past's awareness of itself cannot show.

Some one said: "The dead writers are remote from us because we know so much more than they did." Precisely, and they are that which we know.

I am alive to a usual objection to what is clearly part of my programme for the métier of poetry. The objection is that the doctrine requires a ridiculous amount of erudition (pedantry), a claim which can be rejected by appeal to the lives of poets in any pantheon. It will even be affirmed that much learning deadens or perverts poetic sensibility. While, however, we persist in believing that a poet ought to know as much as will not encroach upon his necessary receptivity and necessary laziness, it is not desirable to confine knowledge to whatever can be put into a useful shape for examinations, drawing-rooms, or the still more pretentious modes of publicity. Some can absorb knowledge, the more tardy must sweat for it. Shakespeare acquired more essential history from Plutarch than most men could from the whole British Museum.

What is to be insisted upon is that the poet must develop or procure the consciousness of the past and that he should continue to develop this consciousness throughout his career.

What happens is a continual surrender of himself as he is at the moment to something which is more valuable. The progress of an artist is a continual self-sacrifice, a continual extinction of personality.

There remains to define this process of depersonalization and its relation to the sense of tradition. It is in this depersonalization that art may be said to approach the condition of science. I, therefore, invite you to consider, as a suggestive analogy, the action which takes place when a bit of finely filiated platinum is introduced into a chamber containing oxygen and sulphur dioxide.

II

Honest criticism and sensitive appreciation are directed not upon the poet but upon the poetry. If we attend to the confused cries of the newspaper critics and the susurrus of popular repetition that follows, we shall hear the names of poets in great numbers; if we seek not Blue-book knowledge but the enjoyment of poetry, and ask for a poem, we shall seldom find it. I have tried to point out the importance of the relation of the poem to other poems by other authors, and suggested the conception of poetry as a living whole of all the poetry that has ever been written. The other aspect of this Impersonal theory of poetry is the relation of the poem to its author. And I hinted, by an analogy, that the mind of the mature poet differs from that of the immature one not precisely in any valuation of "personality," not being necessarily more interesting, or having "more to say," but rather by being a more finely perfected medium in which special, or very varied, feelings are at liberty to enter into new combinations.

The analogy was that of the catalyst. When the two gases previously mentioned are mixed in the presence of a filament of platinum, they form sulphurous acid. This combination takes place only if the platinum is present; nevertheless the newly formed acid contains no trace of platinum, and the platinum itself is apparently unaffected; has remained inert, neutral, and unchanged. The mind of the poet is the shred of platinum. It may partly or exclusively operate upon the experience of the man himself; but, the more perfect the artist, the more completely separate in him will be the man who suffers and the mind which creates; the more perfectly will the mind digest and transmute the passions which are its material.

The experience, you will notice, the elements which enter the presence of the transforming catalyst, are of two kinds: emotions and feelings. The effect of a work of art upon the person who enjoys it is an experience different in kind from any experience not of art. It may be formed out of one emotion, or may be a combination of several; and various feelings, inhering for the writer in particular words or phrases or images, may be added to compose the final result. Or great poetry may be made without the direct use of any emotion whatever: composed out of feelings solely. Canto XV of the Inferno (Brunetto Latini) is a working up of the emotion evident in the situation; but the effect, though single as that of any work of art, is obtained by considerable complexity of detail. The last quatrain gives an image, a feeling attaching to an image, which "came," which did not develop simply out of what precedes, but which was probably in suspension in the poet's mind until the proper combination arrived for it to add itself to. The poet's mind is in fact a receptacle for seizing and storing up numberless feelings, phrases, images, which remain there until all the particles which can unite to form a new compound are present together.

If you compare several representative passages of the greatest poetry you see how great is the variety of types of combination, and also how completely any semi-ethical criterion of "sublimity" misses the mark. For it is not the "greatness," the intensity, of the emotions, the components, but the intensity of the artistic process, the pressure, so to speak, under which the fusion takes place, that counts. The episode of Paolo and Francesca employs a definite emotion, but the intensity of the poetry is something quite different from whatever intensity in the supposed experience it may give the impression of. It is no more intense, furthermore, than Canto XXVI, the voyage of Ulysses, which has not the direct dependence upon an emotion. Great variety is possible in the process of transmutation of emotion: the murder of Agamemnon, or the agony of Othello, gives an artistic effect apparently closer to a possible original than the scenes from Dante. In the Agamemnon, the artistic emotion approximates to the emotion of an actual spectator; in Othello to the emotion of the protagonist himself. But the difference between art and the event is always absolute; the combination which is the murder of Agamemnon is probably as complex as that which is the voyage of Ulysses. In either case there has been a fusion of elements. The ode of Keats contains a number of feelings which have nothing particular to do with the nightingale, but which the nightingale, partly, perhaps, because of its attractive name, and partly because of its reputation, served to bring together.

The point of view which I am struggling to attack is perhaps related to the metaphysical theory of the substantial unity of the soul: for my meaning is, that the poet has, not a "personality" to express, but a particular medium, which is only a medium and not a personality, in which impressions and experiences combine in peculiar and unexpected ways. Impressions and experiences which are important for the man may take no place in the poetry, and those which become important in the poetry may play quite a negligible part in the man, the personality.

I will quote a passage which is unfamiliar enough to be regarded with fresh attention in the light—or darkness—of these observations:

And now methinks I could e'en chide myself
For doating on her beauty, though her death
Shall be revenged after no common action.
Does the silkworm expend her yellow labours
For thee? For thee does she undo herself?
Are lordships sold to maintain ladyships
For the poor benefit of a bewildering minute?
Why does yon fellow falsify highways,
And put his life between the judge's lips,
To refine such a thing—keeps horse and men
To beat their valours for her? . . . [1]

In this passage (as is evident if it is taken in its context) there is a combination of positive and negative emotions: an intensely strong attraction toward beauty and an equally intense fascination by the ugliness which is contrasted with it and which destroys it. This balance of contrasted emotion is in the dramatic situation to which the speech is pertinent, but that situation alone is inadequate to it. This is, so to speak, the structural emotion, provided by the drama. But the whole effect, the dominant tone, is due to the fact that a number of floating feelings, having an affinity to this

The Bizarchives

Weird Tales of Monsters, Magic and Machines

Publishers of Strange Fiction
TheBizarchives.com

emotion by no means superficially evident, have combined with it to give us a new art emotion.

It is not in his personal emotions, the emotions provoked by particular events in his life, that the poet is in any way remarkable or interesting. His particular emotions may be simple, or crude, or flat. The emotion in his poetry will be a very complex thing, but not with the complexity of the emotions of people who have very complex or unusual emotions in life. One error, in fact, of eccentricity in poetry is to seek for new human emotions to express; and in this search for novelty in the wrong place it discovers the perverse. The business of the poet is not to find new emotions, but to use the ordinary ones and, in working them up into poetry, to express feelings which are not in actual emotions at all. And emotions which he has never experienced will serve his turn as well as those familiar to him. Consequently, we must believe that "emotion recollected in tranquillity" is an inexact formula. For it is neither emotion, nor recollection, nor, without distortion of meaning, tranquillity. It is a concentration, and a new thing resulting from the concentration, of a very great number of experiences which to the practical and active person would not seem to be experiences at all; it is a concentration which does not happen consciously or of deliberation. These experiences are not "recollected," and they finally unite in an atmosphere which is "tranquil" only in that it is a passive attending upon the event. Of course this is not quite the whole story. There is a great deal, in the writing of poetry, which must be conscious and deliberate. In fact, the bad poet is usually unconscious where he ought to be conscious, and conscious where he ought to be unconscious. Both errors tend to make him "personal." Poetry is not a turning loose of emotion, but an escape from emotion; it is not the expression of personality, but an escape from personality. But, of course, only those who have personality and emotions know what it means to want to escape from these things.

III

δ δε νους ισως Θειοτερον τι και απαθες εστιν [2]

This essay proposes to halt at the frontier of metaphysics or mysticism, and confine itself to such practical conclusions as can be applied by the responsible person interested in poetry. To divert interest from the poet to the poetry is a laudable aim: for it would conduce to a juster estimation of actual poetry, good and bad. There are many people who appreciate the expression of sincere emotion in verse, and there is a smaller number of people who can appreciate technical excellence. But very few know when there is an expression of significant emotion, emotion which has its life in the poem and not in the history of the poet. The emotion of art is impersonal. And the poet cannot reach this impersonality without surrendering himself wholly to the work to be done. And he is not likely to know what is to be done unless he lives in what is not merely the present, but the present moment of the past, unless he is conscious, not of what is dead, but of what is already living.

[1] From Cyril Tourner's play *Revenger's Tragedy* (1607).

[2] "Presumably the mind is something more divine, and is unaffected." Aristotle, *On the Soul,* 408b.

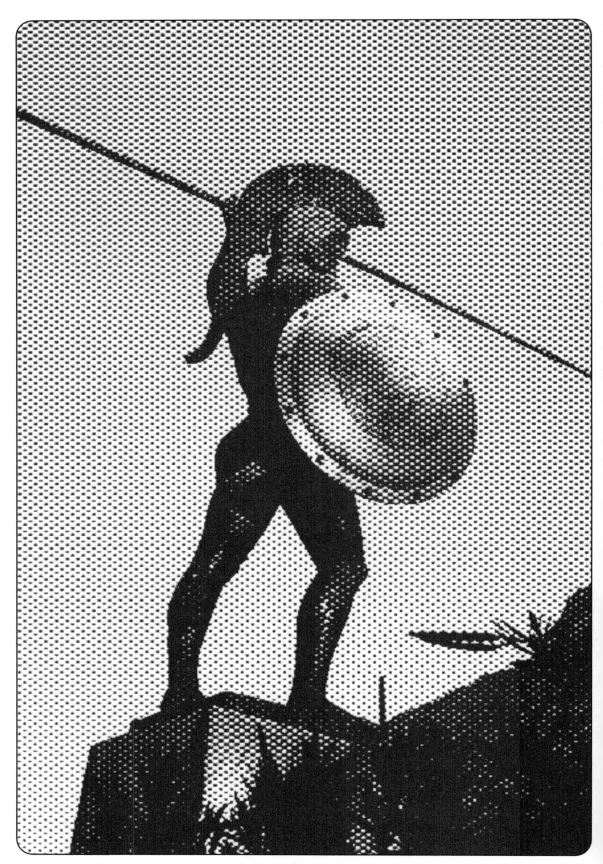

FREE MEN AND SLAVES

essay **BY SCOTT LOCKLIN**

We would do well to remember that slavery is a mindset as much as a physical state, says SCOTT LOCKLIN

It's little remarked upon, but the vast majority of people alive today are descended from slaves and peasants. Most of these people remain emotional slaves and peasants.

Nietzsche was the last prominent scholar to make such statements, though most misunderstood him. Nietzsche was what I like to describe as a sort of modern Ancient Greek philosopher. He was a philologist; a classicist. His actual philosophy is something like what I'd imagine a pre-Socratic such as Heraclitus might be if he were a Polish Lutheran with poor digestion, writing in Wilhelmine German. The pre-Socratics were the philosophy of the Hellenes at their peak. Socrates was a sort of Jonathan Rawls. The Hellenes even well past their prime were mostly concerned with what we now call moral philosophy rather than analytic philosophy: how to live.

Nietzsche's admonition of slave morality is precisely the type of thing an Ancient Greek philosopher would say, and should be taken in a similar spirit. Recognizing that most of the people around you are spiritual and mental slaves, descended from spiritual and mental and ultimately actual slaves is important in understanding the condition of The Current Year.

The peasant/slave reaction to saying this, is of course, cattle-like fear and loathing. Most people think slavery consists in some sort of S&M accoutrements, like in the TV shows. The reality is, slaves through most of human history didn't require shackles to keep them fixed in place, and they slept in beds and performed work which was normal for their times. Slavery was, and is, very much a state of mind.

Some of the slaves of ancient times were that way because they were born to it. Others became slaves through conquest or debt. The actual conditions of slavery were not generally distinguishable from the life of a free man: slaves worked in agriculture, but also as artificers, clerks, engineers, bankers, even high viziers in some government roles. Slaves were allowed to hold some forms of property, had religious liberty within the household cult, and while they were allowed families, they were not allowed a lineage: they had no family name. Much like most men living today, they have a last name, but generally have no idea as to their lineage past their grandparents.

Some of the Greeks thought certain people were made by nature to be slaves: people who had no capacity for foresight or self-discipline. Aristotle said that unlike animals or very young children, the slave could understand reasoning; he just couldn't do it himself. Essentially, Aristotle was describing the current year NPC, which is probably why the meme stings them so greatly. As he put it in book one of *Politics*, "For the slave has no deliberative faculty at all."

Classical-era slaves were forbidden many things available to free men: for example, they were forbidden gymnastics, weightlifting and wrestling in Athens. These sorts of exercises make the slave more dangerous as they build thumos ("spiritedness", roughly) and character. Even gladiators were fed a diet consisting of legumes, breads and porridge – the kind of slop the sinister docker-pants-wearing goons in WEF meetings would like the whole world to eat along with cockroach tapenade.

Xenophon in his *Education of Cyrus* describes how Cyrus kept the conquered peoples in bondage after conquest. Quite simply, he made them into sybaritic degenerates: the pleasures of the slave. Have fun, don't exercise. Here: have some more wine. Don't experience too much hardship: that would be unpleasant. Slaves were portrayed in the arts as timid, dumb and cowardly. More or less like suburban office dwellers, the types of people who publicly and immediately forgive the killers of their children.

Tyrants and tyrannies love slaves and slavish subjects. Nero famously gave slaves the right to take their masters to court. This wasn't some prototypical love of human dignity or "civil rights" – through perhaps it was done for similar reasons. It was explicitly done to reduce the status of free men. They were all slaves to a tyrant such as Nero. Aristotle knew:

"Again, the evil practices of the last and worst form of democracy are all found in tyrannies. Such are the power given to women in their families in the hope that they will inform against their husbands, and the license which is allowed to slaves in order that they may betray their masters; for slaves and women do not conspire against tyrants; and they are of course friendly to tyrannies and also to democracies, since under them they have a good time. "

The history of modernity is to a certain extent is the mobilization of historical peasant and slave classes for other tasks. Past mobilization was done for warfare and industrial production. The dipshits in power (mostly clerks and slaves themselves, all stupid) now think automation is so well developed, the mass should be back to overt slavery and peonage.

The greatest fear of our enemies is that large numbers of free men will stop acting like slaves. Hence their shrill terror of men with the relatively trivial self-discipline to exercise with weights, stop masturbating, tan their balls or declare they won't eat the bugs. The spirit of not being a slave: to die rather than submit – the virtues of yesteryear crush the life out of the flabby eunuch class.

I'll let Aristotle have the last word:

> **Slaves were portrayed in the arts as timid, dumb and cowardly. More or less like suburban office dwellers, the types of people who publicly and immediately forgive the killers of their children**

"…the tyrant should lop off those who are too high; he must put to death men of spirit; he must not allow common meals, clubs, education, and the like; he must be upon his guard against anything which is likely to inspire either courage or confidence among his subjects; he must prohibit literary assemblies or other meetings for discussion, and he must take every means to prevent people from knowing one another (for acquaintance begets mutual confidence)… In short, he should practice these and the like Persian and barbaric arts, which all have the same object. A tyrant should also endeavor to know what each of his subjects says or does, and should employ spies, like the 'female detectives' at Syracuse, and the eavesdroppers whom Hiero was in the habit of sending to any place of resort or meeting; for the fear of informers prevents people from speaking their minds, and if they do, they are more easily found out. Another art of the tyrant is to sow quarrels among the citizens; friends should be embroiled with friends, the people with the notables, and the rich with one another. Also he should impoverish his subjects; he thus provides against the maintenance of a guard by the citizen and the people, having to keep hard at work, are prevented from conspiring. … Another practice of tyrants is to multiply taxes, after the manner of Dionysius at Syracuse, who contrived that within five years his subjects should bring into the treasury their whole property. The tyrant is also fond of making war in order that his subjects may have something to do and be always in want of a leader."

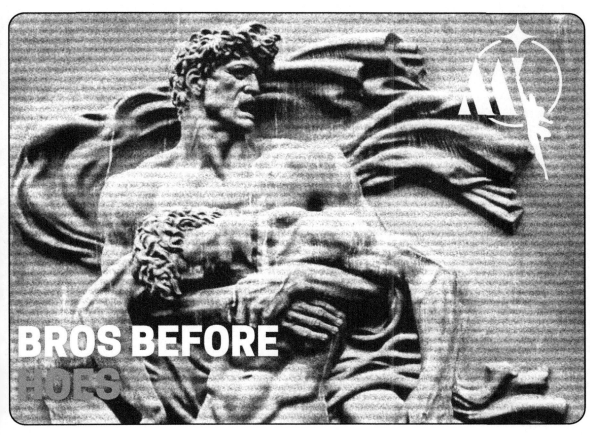

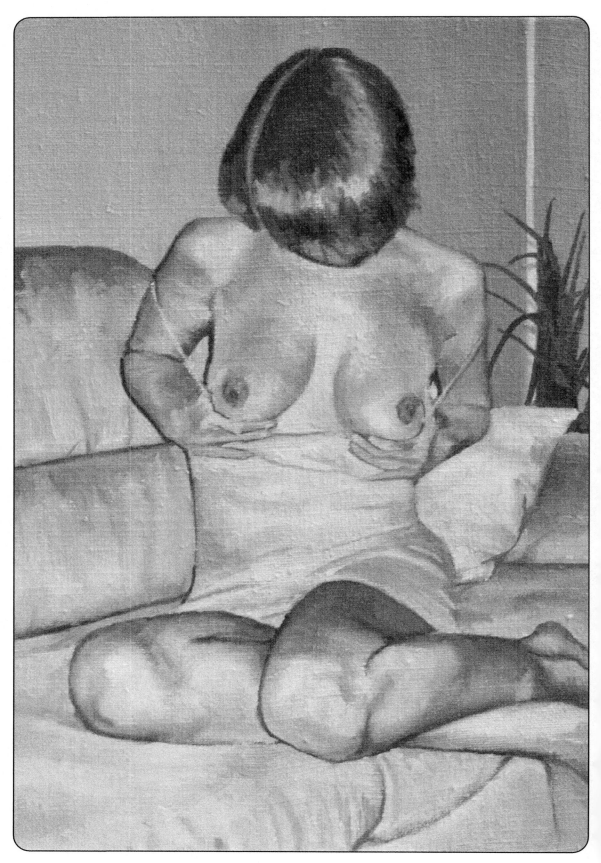

A STRANGE BEAUTY

art **BY ALEXANDER ADAMS**

> The beautiful is always strange. I do not mean that it is coldly, deliberately strange, for in that case it would be a monstrosity that had jumped the rails of life. I mean that it always contains a touch of strangeness, of simple, unpremeditated and unconscious strangeness, and that it is this touch of strangeness that gives it its particular quality as Beauty.
>
> CHARLES BAUDELAIRE

In the year 2000, I started to make the Square Nudes, a series of paintings of nudes on square-format canvases. These nudes would be based on amateur photographs; they would be prosaic, compromised, flattened by harsh light, awkwardly cropped, badly composed. In pictorial and aesthetic terms, they would be crude. I don't mean ugly – although many of the paintings would become tender paintings of ugliness – because there would be beautiful paintings and beautiful subjects. The art would be animated by an uninhibited attitude of a sexual underworld, as stark as it was compelling, something brutishly direct. Most of the photos came from contact magazines, where people advertised for sexual partners.

The aim was to make nude paintings that could not have been made at any other time. These Square Nudes would make would be conditioned by modernity. The trappings would be domestic, banal and contemporary – sagging velveteen sofas, clamshell mobile phones, cheap lingerie, Ikea furniture, strongly patterned carpets. The bodies would also be compromised by modernity. They would be overweight, tattooed, pierced, spray-tanned and with pubic hair modified, as well as some subjects being muscular, slim or athletic. I found myself fascinated by photographs that, although aimed at appealing to others, seemed hopelessly unflattering. Were my standards awry or were these images intended to be squalid? Were these images made to be aggressively, unrelentingly obscene? I did not paint any images of sexual acts, because these seemed to me to distractingly primal, short-circuiting the possibility of disinterested appreciation through the generation of an instinctive visceral attraction or repulsion within the audience.

In the source images, I kept seeing shades of figure paintings by Pierre Bonnard, Edgar Degas and Walter Sickert, no doubt because I am an artist and my memory automatically noticed and compared these photos to those paintings. The project seemed an idle occupation, as I could not imagine any gallery exhibiting the art I was making. It was simply too explicit and tawdry. So, I was painting for my own satisfaction, documenting a cross-section of the adult population who chose to expose their bodies but not their faces. (Contact magazines tended to conceal the faces, which added a dimension of modern anonymity to these nudes.) I interspersed the series with paintings of interiors, which acted as a form of punctuation, relieving the viewer from the unending sequence of genitals and coquetry. The paintings of sinks referred to bodily functions indirectly. The shoddy sinks and public-house urinals became mundane counterparts (even symbolic stand-ins) to the bodies I painted.

As I worked, I could not decide what my responses were to the paintings I made. I found them funny and absurd, yet some figures I painted were undeniably attractive; I developed a protective, paternalistic attitude to the subjects. This happens when you make art. You develop a sympathy with the subjects, even if you consider them ugly or repugnant. When you concentrate and document, you start to lose your distance and pretensions to moral superiority (actual or false). If you stare at a thing long enough, you begin to empathise, forming a peculiar bond. It is the human condition, perhaps. I did not see as attractive the bodies that were elderly, ugly, fat or unsympathetically modified by tattoo or piercing, but I felt compassion, even sadness, towards the subjects. The more faithful I attempted to be in my task of compiling a pictorial encyclopaedia of the contemporary human form in Europe of the 1990s and 2000s, the more my distance from these subjects evaporated. I became deeply ambivalent about the art I was making and my view of the subjects.

Looking back on this series of about 250 paintings (some of which were published in a textless book in 2005, entitled *Noctes*) – and which ended roughly around 2014 – I am still unclear about what I achieved, if anything. Some of the paintings trouble me with their rawness; others seem to have acquired the mantle of a classical nude from ancient Greece or a rococo painting of a court concubine. Although the paintings were made to neutrally record, they also celebrate by raising to the level of fine art the most compromising and crudest of images.

Is the best of contemporary art an artist asking himself questions and hoping to understand himself and the world through the process of working, rather than constructing definitive coherent statements? I used to think that. There seemed something utterly modern in this anomie, this sense of being cut adrift from the certainties of tradition, this lack of centre, this acceptance of the ugly, compromised and squalid alongside the beautiful and correct. Maybe that is truly what modernity consists of and that is what I now reject. Today, I see such relativism and tolerance as a manifestation of society-wide conditioning, from which I was not immune.

The modernity I was painting was not just in the bodies and domestic settings: it was within myself. I was a painter willing to record and re-present these extreme images without condemnation and even without commentary. In a pre-modern era, could any artist have worked in such a way with images considered so graphic, obscene and degrading? I don't know. Viewing this series at a distance, I am coming to understand myself better now. When I think of these paintings, I cannot help but see myself at work on them: unconsciously rejecting my repugnance, overcoming doubts and making images anyway. I am not sure if I still am that artist or that man. I present the paintings again, without individual comment.

Visit alexanderadams.art. He tweets @ adamsartist

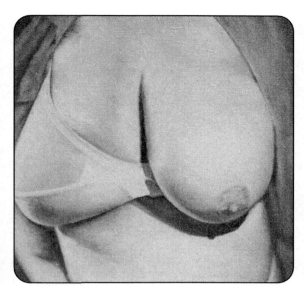
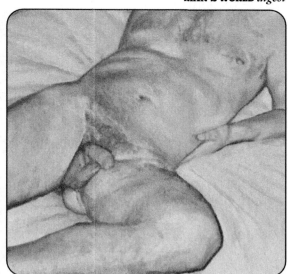
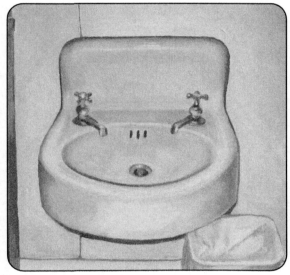
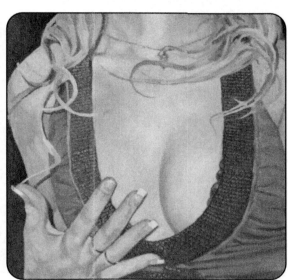
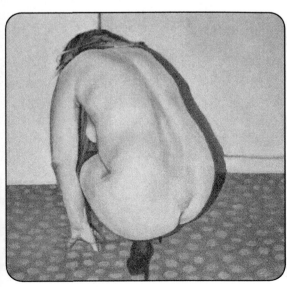
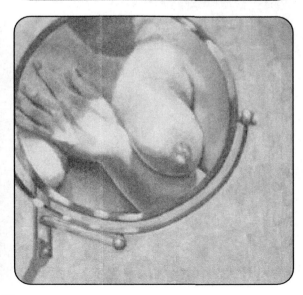

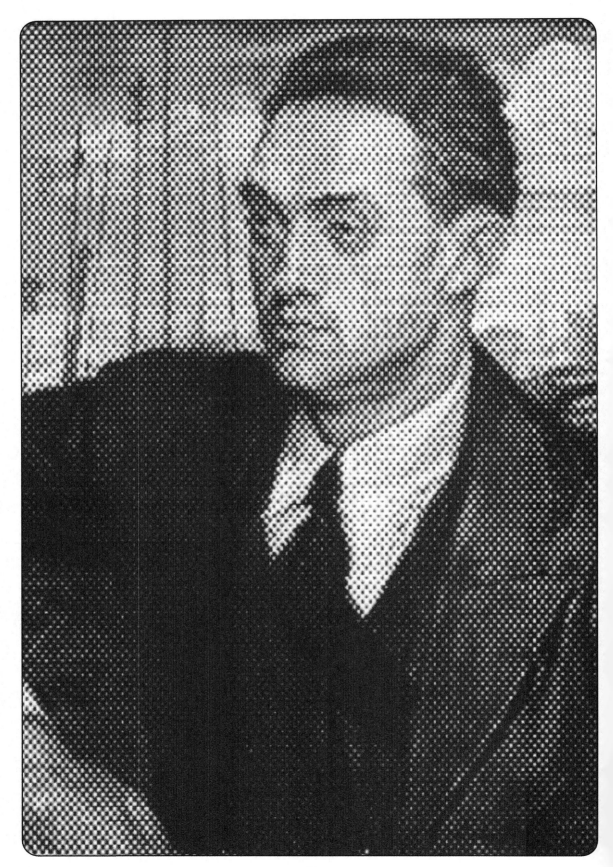

A LETTER FROM A FATHER TO HIS SON

translation BY BRAQUEMART

In this translation by BRAQUEMART (@braquemart1888), French writer Henry de Montherlant (1895-1972) provides a guide for his son and for himself and other men who wish to be a true model and inspire the younger generation. The piece was written in 1935.

The virtues that you will cultivate above all are courage, public-spiritedness, pride, integrity, contempt, disinterestedness, politeness, gratitude, and, in general, all that is understood by the word generosity.

Moral courage, which has such good press, is an easy virtue chiefly for him who does not pay any consideration to opinion. If one does not have it, to acquire it is a matter of will, which is to say an easy matter. On the contrary, if one does not have physical courage, to acquire it is a matter of hygiene, which is outside the framework that I have laid out for myself here.

Public-spiritedness and patriotism are one and the same, if the patriotism is worthy of the name. You are from a country where there is patriotism in fits and starts, and public-spiritedness, never; or public-spiritedness is considered ridiculous. I say to you: "If you are a patriot, be so seriously", as I would say to you: "If you are a Catholic, be so seriously." I do not have great esteem for a man who in wartime valiantly defends the country that he has in peacetime enfeebled by a thousand pinpricks. Do not require that your country be invaded for you to treat it well. Conduct yourself as decently in peace as in war, if you love the peace.

Vanity, which rules the world, is a ridiculous sentiment. Arrogance, well-founded, adds nothing to merit; when I hear talk of a "beautiful arrogance," I become pensive. Unfounded, it is ridiculous even to itself. The only superiority of arrogance to vanity is that vanity waits for everything, and arrogance waits for nothing; arrogance does not need to be nourished, it is passionately fond of sobriety. Halfway between vanity and arrogance, you will choose pride.

Integrity is this and that, and besides it is a good thing. It obtains all that cunning obtains, at less cost, at less risk, and with less time lost.

Disinterestedness has only the merit of extracting you from the vulgar, but it does so for certain. Every time that you, being able to take, do not take, you will give to yourself one hundred and one thousand times more than you would have given by taking. Out of all the opportunities from which you will not wish to benefit, you will construct for yourself a cathedral of diamond in the invisible world. Contemporary France has created a certain number of truly obscene words, among which is gate-crashing. Do not gate-crash, be it in the most humble domain, for that goes from the humble to the great.

Contempt is part of esteem. One is capable of contempt to the degree that one is capable of esteem. The excellent reasons that we have to despise. He who does not despise the bad, or the low, compromises with it. And of what worth is esteem that does not know how to despise? I have always thought that it is possible to found something on contempt; now I know what: morality. It is not arrogance that despises; it is virtue. Much will also be forgiven to him who will have despised much. And again I add this: that it is not necessary to not be despicable in order to despise.

There is no serious hatred that does not contain contempt. For example, I do not hate the Germans, because I do not despise them.

One of the signs of French decline is that she would no longer be capable of contempt.

Politeness, because its absence spoils everything. In the world of today, where politeness will very soon be even rarer than virtue, we will come to the point where some will end by judging that bad education equals bad action. You will always give politeness first, before knowing whether it will be given to you, and you will see to it chiefly with regard to the humble. If it is not given to you, you will break with those people, whatever the interests or the passions involved between you and them may be, and whatever their quality or their merit may be. And you will notice that extreme politeness is as necessary among friends as among strangers: the absence of politeness, with a friend, impairs and then destroys a friendship just as surely as a more dazzling mistake. Politeness will surround your eyes, for it requires a great nervous expenditure. But one cannot do without it.

As a general rule, you will remember to always caution the humble when they do not expect it and to remain reserved with the great. Kindness with the humble, indulgence with the middling, vigilance with the great. Without forgetting that as much charity is necessary with respect to the great as with respect to the humble.

Gratitude is a feeling so contrary to nature that, if you do not take great care, this feeling very much risks escaping you. A person with something of vitality does not care at all whether or not others show him gratitude. But do not count on such vitality.

If you have these virtues, the rest is not as important. It matters little, for example, that you believe in God, or not. You can think however will seem good to you on this matter.

It matters little that you love or do not love your fellow-man. But do not seek after his love. First, because he who gives you his love takes away your liberty. Second, because to seek to please is the most slippery slope for heading straight to the lowest level. We must take from women, lest we limit ourselves in being too masculine, much of the instinct proper to their sex. But, by God! not that one.

It matters little that you yield or do not to sensual pleasure. You will hear it said that pleasure is incompatible with spirituality, charity, good health, etc. This is an illusion. A sufficiently full and balanced nature manages all that and is satisfied. These are passions that it is equal to guiding, that's all. "God knows that you cannot stop yourself from thinking about women."(Koran.) But it is in this domain above all that you must have deportment. Take care to tolerate nothing from women that would make you rear coming from a man. The happiness that a being gives you does not create for it rights over you. To maintain this idea is not always easy, and all the less because we must reconcile it with the great gratitude that whoever has given us pleasure merits.

Many of the actions that common morality takes for innocent condemn a man without recourse. But lying, murder, theft, the pillage of war do not necessarily condemn a man. He can commit them and retain the qualities of superiority. The life of many men is worth no more than the life of a gudgeon. Theft often has excuses. Lying often does less bad than the truth; contrary to common opinion, one can very well lie to those whom one loves the most: you have lied to me, I have lied to you, and I will lie to you yet. Obviously, on all that, you will not make me say what I do not say.

Here are many indifferent things. What is essential is loftiness. It will take the place of everything for you. In it I include detachment, for how can one maintain loftiness without detaching oneself? It will be fatherland enough for you, if you have no other. It will take the place of the fatherland for you, the day that the other fails you. One must be enamored with loftiness, for, in being so, one falls much and more. What will happen, then, if one is not so!

I return to the virtue of contempt, since, as I have told you, it is unknown to our compatriots. "Heliogabalus did not wish to have children, out of fear that that he would only receive ones of honest morals."(Lampride.) I am annoyed to feel myself in disagreement with a head of State, but, if anything had stopped me from having a son, it would have been, on the contrary, the fear that he would not have had honest morals. By "honest morals" I understand above all that quality of a being, by grace of which the bad disgusts him like a vulgarity. We see often enough boys of excellent environments, students of great schools or others, cornered in stories of narcotics, of prostitutes, of shady people and things. They lacked that quality, which would have made it so that they had only to see these people, and without the moral sense intervening, they would have known that with respect to them it would be possible to have only one rule of conduct: that of having nothing in common with them. They lacked repugnance; they lacked contempt. It was a baffling thing for me, and gravely sad, to see what sorts of people young French officers, in the colonies, allowed themselves to be surrounded by. I take officers as an example, because to shock under uniform is to shock doubly. These people were filthy; the first glance at them sufficed for me to lose my temper. For, not only did they not have that effect on young men that we take for that which is better in French society, but these young men took pleasure in their contact. We learn next the classic intrigue of the lieutenant and the spy, or the lieutenant who kills himself for a prostitute. None of such would have occurred if these boys, before these women, had had that sort of quivering that one calls contempt. When one of them gets himself into a filthy story, before even having thought of him: "He is a fool"⊠ which is always the case ⊠ I think: "This is a boy who had no quality." If, on a jury, I heard a father answer the question: "Why did you kill your son?"⊠ "Because he had become a loafer", it seems to me that I would vote for acquittal. But this disposition is not exactly that in which justice is dispensed today.

I was just brought carnations and roses that someone whom I do not like sent me. I remove their frames with care, as if I were removing a pin from the body of a butterfly. That rose, enamored of its long stem, how good it feels! Surely the angel Gabriel took it between his fingers. I breathe it, while holding its corolla in both palms, as the heaviest of goblets, or as a bird that one would retain without squeezing. If there is a worm at the bottom, and which I have allowed to enter my nostrils, frankly, God help me! This evening she will have no more perfume; I will have completely inhaled all her perfume. I will sleep on it while holding it against my chest, with its long stem, like a king, in his tomb, his scepter. But it is chiefly in electric lighting that one must see it. Nothing equals the fire, the vigor, the brilliance, the all-powerful youth of the colors of carnations and roses when electricity abruptly illuminates them in the middle of the night. I will send you a third of this basket of flowers, while keeping the rest for myself.

I never understood that a man is to show his hearth, not his friends, not his manner of working, not his manner of praying ⊠ in a word, his life. Har'm, say the Muslims, and this expression collects also all that they love. However I would tell you less: "Be secretive", rather than: "Have the ability to be so." In moral life, that which is hidden is more intense, as, in clothing of poor quality, the fabric, under the reverse, conserves a more vivid color. A man who does not know how to guard a secret is judged. And remember that the difficulty is not to conceal from nine others, but to conceal it also from the tenth.

You will have a reasonable gentleness with respect to animals, for all the reasons that are usually given, but chiefly because you will often find among them more nobility and more justice than among men. Each time that you will have resisted needlessly killing an animal, or needlessly annoying it, you will have done well.

The same with regard to objects. Each time that you will have resisted plucking a flower, pissing in clear water, needlessly breaking a branch, etc., you will have done well. When there is no certain merit in it (and that is not certain), you will at least have avoided a vulgar gesture.

I caution you against fear of opinion. Woe to him who wishes not to be slandered! A man who knows what he is worth, when he sees himself disregarded, slandered, in good faith or not, has only one feeling: surprise. There are plenty of other things that give him disgust and hate. Contrive some periods of disrepute; alternate them with periods in which you are esteemed. When you will have perceived that they have exactly the same flavor, you will have taken a good step toward a sane view of things. And then, when people do not think well of you, it is then that there is merit in being virtuous. There is absolutely no merit in being so when we are showered with praise; they gradually take the virtues that they attribute to you.

On this matter you say to me: "How to reconcile the point of honor, which seems to imply the importance given to opinion, with this last disdain for opinion?" Oh, my dear, that is part of your gymnastic. You would not wish that I give you everything cut and dry.

I caution you against ambition. It is good that I do this ahead of time, for it is a passion that is part of the stupidity of the young. It was not before twenty-eight that I discovered that ambition was a bourgeois passion. Obviously, you can amuse yourself with this feeling, like with any other, in the manner of a pastime.

I caution you against excess callousness. I caution you against excess will. Take care! An immense part of the energy that men expend is expended for nothing. Give yourself only in earnest. And that will be easier for you, if you recall that a person like yourself is not too attached to what he does. He who says eagerness says plebeian (of the soul, obviously).

There is no suffering the sting of which you cannot blunt by imagining how it could be worse. Consciousness of vexations is rapidly eliminated in a man who has good circulation. I caution you nevertheless, as a reminder, against useless suffering (everything that I am going to say to you about this is said concerning moral suffering). Happiness is a considerably more noble and refined state than suffering: when humanity had a sane mind, the gods that she created she made happy. It is not in depths of pain that I have seen anything at all: there one is encircled by a wall of stupidity. It is from the summits of bliss that I have seen that which I had to see. That from that time men rarely win happiness: they are not worthy enough of it. Lacking it, they slander it. If nature wished anything, it would not be suffering that it would wish; it is only to see how people who suffer become mean, ugly, go to pieces, sometimes lose their judgement, etc. Every time that you will hear talk of the primacy of suffering, you will be able to wager that you are faced with a vulgar spirit: suffering is the small luxury of people of mediocre quality. It is for him who would wish to have others believe that he is the most unhappy and the most uneasy, like these young girls whom I heard conversing one day: "You know, I cry loudly." "Me, I cry more loudly than you. If I cry, everyone can hear me from the street." Almost all people are so: they want to be heard from the street. The majority of moral sufferings are sufferings that they entirely create for themselves, without reason; not only are they unfounded, they are also useless. Ah! physical suffering is otherwise more respectable. Take then just as much moral suffering as is necessary for the richness and diversity of your interior life, but be happy, in remaining proper; one must feel oneself at ease in nature. And, when you will be happy, know that you are so, and be not ashamed to acknowledge a state so worthy of esteem.

When you will have become this rare exemplary human, which alone will justify my having made you, then without doubt will the time have come for you to have yourself killed for the quarrels of a civilization to which you do not feel yourself bound.

If not for you, of the past and the future, it would still be the future which interested me the least. But in being born you created for me the future; you made me its prisoner. It is in the nature of things that one day of this future you will turn against me. In the age in which I will conclude my life, it will be obvious to you that I was overpraised, and that in reality I was an imbecile. It will be strangers who flower my grave, not you. Do not disquiet yourself too much on account of this sham "wretched feeling". I will not be too disquieted about it myself. It is deeply indifferent

> **There is no suffering the sting of which you cannot blunt by imagining how it could be worse. Consciousness of vexations is rapidly eliminated in a man who has good circulation**

to me that you love me or not, and I would be ashamed to have the desire for it; your sympathy will be all that is necessary. I am much attached to you: I am content with this feeling. I love lemonade. I do not need lemonade to love me.

One day, then, you may say to me that the advice that I have given you is not suitable for a modern man. Certainly: the virtues that I ask of you are the most injurious to him who wishes "to succeed" (always these obscene words) in the modern world. But I did not make you so that you could be a modern man, but just a man.

To which you may say to me that it is not that which will give you bread, the day when you will have the misfortune of having to win your bread. ("the misfortune": for, as you know, I hate work. The religion of the Christians saw well, which made of it the great Punishment; which wished, in the Middle Ages, that the perfectly spiritual man live on alms rather than work.) To which I will reply that you will always find ways of winning your bread; it is not advice on that matter that you will lack, nor the examples: people have only that in their heads. But I, I will have given you the means of eating and drinking to the idea that you will have improved yourself. And that can take the place of part of your bread for you.

I am distracted from what I was going to write you by a charming greyhound that is passing in front of the garden. The fur of its rear tendons is entirely pink, and translucent. To think that it carries everywhere with him these two immarcescible gemstones!

One can hear streams, dogs, and bees. All that penetrates what I write to you. I express myself poorly: that cannot penetrate it, since they are one and the same.

One day, you may say to me that men are worthy of neither that kindness, nor these sacrifices, nor that generosity, nor even justice. That is possible. But it is not for them that you will have had these virtues, it is for you. You will say to me that there is no cause that could be worth dying for. That is quite likely. "What then! Is one to die, is one to suffer for a cause in which one believes only halfway?" But it is not for that cause that one suffers and one dies. It is for the idea that that suffering and that death give you of yourself. It is necessary to be irrational, my friend, but it is not necessary to be a dupe. No pity for dupes.

With all that, you will have your approbation and mine. It will suffice you. For, just as you do not expect your virtues to be useful for anything, in the same way, and even more powerfully, will you not expect that it take you into consideration. On the contrary, I will say to you what the Stoics said to the sage: you will be sacrificed to it totally. For each of your "good" deeds you will be automatically punished. He who is brave is killed, he who seeks justice is treated with indifference, he who marries as a point of honor ruins his life. Liberality impoverishes, mercy emboldens the mean, sincerity gives them arms, firmness of soul prevents others from taking your troubles seriously, self-mastery is taken for bloodlessness, reason for cowardice, modesty for incapacity, forgiveness for consent to their wrongs. And it is very difficult to wish to be bad to men on that account, when one sees that the unfailing return for being happy and esteemed is to systematically smother all the movements of one's conscience and heart. Of the diverse means that you have today of making yourself hated by your compatriots, the most sure is to have elevated sentiments. All that will put you in their favor they will return against you. They will not hate you, so much as they will attribute to your actions the only motives that make them act themselves, that is paltry motives; they will hate you as soon as they suspect other motives. They would prefer that you be their tormenter than their benefactor, provided that, as their tormenter, they would feel you to be at their level; you will find in the society that surrounds you a universal complacency, except with respect to that which is different. They will scoff at you and disparage you, and at this sign you will understand that you are on the right path. To the degree that you are advised to systematically slide from here to there, some thing that attracts jeering, in order to be really sure that they are scoffing at you, to such a degree is that sign certain. Moreover there is always the pleasure of supplying arms to one's enemies; to this you will quickly take a liking that you will soon no longer be able to do without. This is not to say that it is necessary to be hated. But, the world being as it is, how would an honest man not be proud to inspire that feeling in it?

Will you know how to maintain that state of inferiority in which I seek to place you in the social game? My poor child, you lack covetousness, you lack fury, you lack impudence: how will you make up for that? I seem to see the maliciousness of the world, as the birds do on their boughs, perching on you to make you yield. Your mildness gives me fear. For the sixteen years that you have been on this earth, you have been my wonder: I have never had anything to reproach you for that would have marked enough to leave a trace on me, and the respect that I show you is worthy of that which you have shown me there. Such as you show yourself to me, I see you stripped of all harshness, all evasion, all affectation. One would say that a kind of isolating polish renders you insensitive, without effort on your part, to all that is vile. And the days go by, bringing reasons to corrupt you in handfuls, yet without corrupting you; and I view you as one views a well-born being, that is to say that which is rarest in the world, but also which suffices to justify it, and fearing unceasingly that the idea that I have of you will not crack gradually, because you will have taken a misstep. For all that, it happens that some strangers complain about you. Would you then help me? I have never sought to penetrate your feelings with respect to me; I told you that they matter little to me. But I would like to be sure that far from me you preserve enough rigor to resist, not only that which is bad, but also that which is not made for you. That honesty and that modesty that you carry with you, like the greyhound his two marvelous gemstones, will be more threatened than ever before. By the world, and by you yourself: for you are going to enter that "awkward age" of life, that runs from about the eighteenth to the twenty-eighth year, in which one must almost necessarily be a fool (and it is through foolishness, quite often, that one finds attraction to the vulgarities of the bad). You are in a canoe, that is your newness, on an ocean of excrement, that is the world; it will be a miracle if you do not capsize. And it would then be necessary for me to despise that to which I gave life! To become the equal of those unhappy unconscious ones who are the majority of fathers and mothers! My young boy! But I stop myself, for I sense that I trouble myself when I think too much of what you are for me. And I have better things to do with you, than to love you.

Visit braquemart.substack.com for more exclusive translations of authors including de Montherlant.

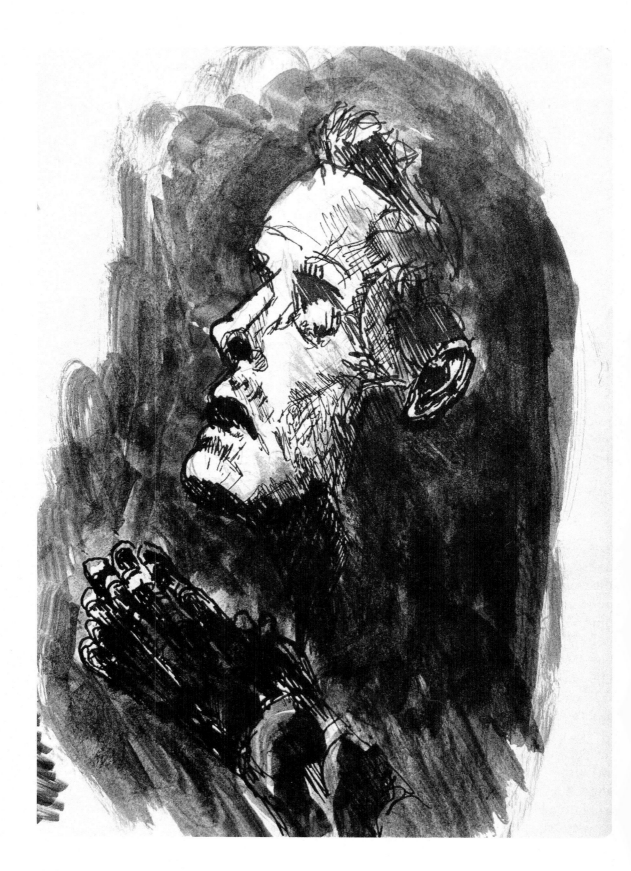

LET'S NOT DECLARE A PANDEMIC AMNESTY

art BY GIO PENNACCHIETTI

As has been noted by one critic, what makes the strange dream worlds of Kafka's writing "so convincingly uncanny", is the way the protagonists "seem to be colluding in their own punishment."

If only the main character in *The Trial* left his house and stopped consenting to such a line of absurd questioning! If only Gregor Samsa stopped internalizing his bug-man state! If only we did not choose to descend into hating family members, or being coerced into unwanted medical decisions! If only. But these questions open up wounds that run deeper than anyone would care to admit in the aftermath of a total shredding of the social fabric. I cannot forgive my government for treating me with contempt and scorn; the dead cannot forgive for the crimes of state-enforced loneliness before death, and the careless and clinical way they were treated after death, denied ritual and the sentiments of families grieving together.

Meet conservative women near you!

We know how frustrating it can be trying to connect with people who don't hold traditional values.

That's why we came up with Right Time, a new dating app that cuts to the chase and puts you in contact with women who want the same things as you do.

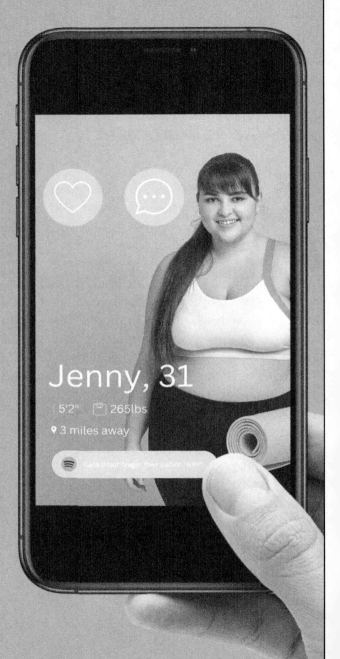

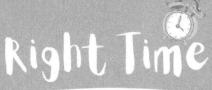

Now is the Right Time for you to step up.

Available from the App Store and Google Play

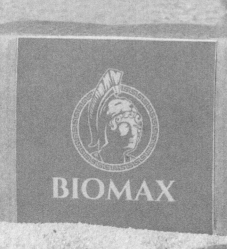

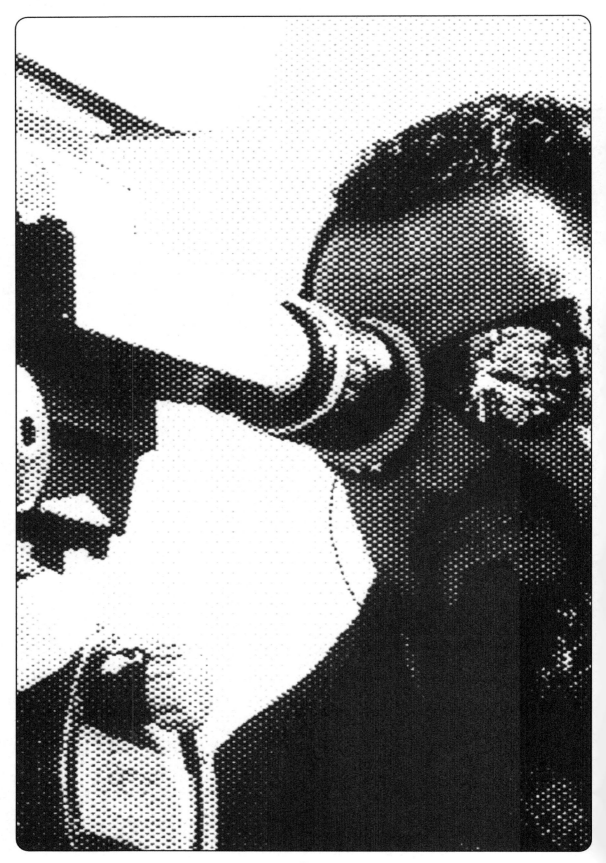

THE RADICAL ARISTOCRAT OF HOLLYWOOD

film **BY YAMNAYANAGE**

The filmmaker John Milius is a throwback to another age not just in film, but also in man's history, says YAMNAYANAGE

Jonathan Bowden said of Nietzsche, "His was an ethical superstructure for a radically aristocratic way of thinking which once existed in the past." If Hollyweird ever had such a man it was John Milius, the man who refused the Hollywood Industrial Complex "norms". A place where ethics are notoriously penumbral, a place that summons demons and thus by nature demands an equally savage spirit to battle against. That spirit sprung out of the abyss in the form of John Milius, a Bronze Age anachronism thundering, inveighing as only a righwing zealot can. "A lot of the principles by which I live were dead before I was born." He smoked cigars inside Warner Brothers's "smoke-free" studios and offices. He refused traditional payment, demanding handguns and a SUV full of illegal Cuban cigars instead. John asserted his radically aristocratic way of living in a world where such philistine and buccaneering impulses were abhorred.

His was an impulse to action. It was the only true sense of being; he did therefore he was. He grabbed the bull by the horns, balls – anything – as long as his fists were clenched tight and he was engaged with life in a way that most men will not even consider a possibility for themselves. His was not a domestic life, but one which subsumed adventure, combat and physical stimulus. Faulkner said, "I believe that man will not merely endure, he will prevail." With over 23 screenwriting credits to his name, most of which howled in the face the radical-left, Milius is a man who did more than prevail. Milius is a man who conquered.

Armed with a writing style heavily influenced by the muscular, Anglo-Saxon prose of Hemingway – terse and direct like a hard right to the jaw – Milius told the stories that he liked to read, steeped deeply in the lore of Homeric hero and hardy frontiersman. His was a type of syntax that once punctuated Hollywood's most memorable scripts, written for the old gods of cinema, but which had fallen from favor. He was the resurrecting voice, which breathed life back into the sleeping giants of violence and vitality. He alone channeled the cold-hearted bastard, who blacked pity's eye and shattered its jaw.

This concept of masculinity and storytelling came from Milius's father. Dad Milius was a WWI vet and Harvard grad who would read John stories of Teddy's "Rough Riders" and James Fenimore Cooper's rugged frontiersman. When John delved into juvenile delinquency, his father sent him to boarding school in Steamboat, CO. Nestled within the Rocky Mountains was a school where John could check out a rifle, a horse and camping gear for the weekend. His naturalist spirit and his ability to write were fostered by a young, unorthodox teacher. Wayne Kakela was a recent Dartmouth grad who traveled the world by motorcycle, participated in biathlons (cross-country skiiing and rifle shooting) and encouraged his male students to engage not only with the great classics but also the great outdoors. While educating them on the likes of Homer, Hemingway, Faulkner and Conrad, he would co-opt their labor, for instance to craft an outdoor sauna.

After high school, John's life purpose remained elusive until he wandered into a film festival while on an "endless summer" trip to Hawaii. It was here that he saw the films of Kurosawa for the first time, and his purpose became clearer. He returned to Southern California and enrolled in film school, a still nascent idea within Hollywood. As luck would have it, he graduated into a box office bear market; James Bond's waifu fantasy *You Only Live Twice* delivered a 25% drop at the box office compared to 1965's *Thunderball* and Hollywood was realizing that Connery's hair piece was now as obvious as their inability to deliver results. Even legendary talents like Director Howard Hawks and John Wayne were doing retreads (*El Dorado*) of their own films, and still couldn't match the box office power of the original (*Rio Bravo*, 1959). The studio old guard, etiolated and out of ideas, were willing to take a gamble on any writer who could help refill their empty coffers.

While Milius did pick up some part time work, it was mostly the NEET life of surf, sun and skanks that earned his full-time attention. While Milius was living in a bomb shelter under his landlord's home, an agent across the street noticed the bombshelter bordello and its nightly cavalcade of bimbo habitues. He told John to give up surfing and sleeping around and get serious. John did not listen. A practicing Pagan, he named his surfboard Odin's Arrow and earned the nickname "Viking Man" for his fearlessness on the sea, his captivating yarns around the fires of beachside barbecues, and his ability to take surf groupie brides. He found an altar at the foot of rolling Southern California pipelines. "It was like a religion… We were all living at an intensity which couldn't be substituted by any drug, or job, or even women."

John's first significant success came in 1970 when he sold his script for *Jeremiah Johnson*. He earned $5,000 for the initial sale, but after being hired, fired, and rehired numerous times he ended up making close to $100,000 in total. With a newly formed mercenary drive to write, he exacted his tribute. Like an Alciabiades of Hollywood, he would hold up productions: if he was writing he'd torment directors, if he was directing he'd terrorize studio heads. The enfant terrible, the gadfly, the agent provocateur, no matter what they called him, he had

> **While Milius was living in a bomb shelter under his landlord's home, an agent across the street noticed the bombshelter bordello and its nightly cavalcade of bimbo habitues**

writing talent and he delivered results.

Millius said, "(Director Sydney) Pollack always looked at me like I was crazy or was going to do something horrible or attack everybody or start gnawing human flesh." It was this Dionysian spirit of chaos and frenzy that undoubtedly fed the crazed ravings of his fully scalped yet vitalistic character, Del Gue:

"These (mountains) here is God's finest sculpturings! And there ain't no laws for the brave ones! And there ain't no asylums for the crazy ones! And there ain't no churches, except for this right here! And there ain't no priests excepting the birds. By God, I are a mountain man, and I'll live 'til an arrow or a bullet finds me."

Yet amidst his thundering, semi-non-sequitur tirades existed the Apollonian spirit of rugged individualism. It was John's firm belief that purity inspired the mountain man's savagery. Their desire for clean water, clear air, and unclaimed space revived long forgotten demands for savagery. It was savagery that asserted their place in that pure terrain. They were the first, and the first must always endure the bloodiest battles if they are to remain.

Embodying that type of ethos kept John constantly embroiled in feuds with the Hollywood elite. Milius saw Jeremiah Johnson and his struggle against the Crow in these terms:

"The feud will go on forever, and it makes both of them bigger and makes them live forever and also kills them. And these are the way all feuds are, the way the Hatfields and the McCoys are, the Capulets and Montagues, and the feuds in Borneo among the Dyaks. When I was making Farewell to the King in Borneo I'd ask the Dayaks, 'What started this feud?' and they'd say, 'It doesn't matter. The feud has been here since the time of God.'"

Milius was fully taken by the romantic notion of holding forth against an adversary, against insurmountable odds that would certainly end in death or at the very least loss of limb or physical function.

***

Milius was in the back of a sedan headed to Palm Springs to meet Frank Sinatra for the second time. In his briefcase was a handgun. Milius's classic Smith and Wesson, four-inch model 29, which he had written into the script for *Dirty Harry*. Sinatra, who was lined up for the Harry Callahan role, had asked Milius to bring "the gat" that he was supposed to use in the film. When Frank saw the gun, after he had laced into his bodyguard for letting it get into his house unannounced (typical CA liberal, some things never change), he picked it up and acted out the famous line then set it back down. "Ooh, it's a big one! Too big." By the time Milius had driven back to LA from Palm Springs, Sinatra had decided he didn't want to be in films anymore.

Now it was between Burt Reynolds and Clint Eastwood, and since Eastwood was younger, they figured he'd be more amiable when it came to doing scenes that Reynolds disliked (i.e. "stunts"). The studio took Eastwood off *Jeremiah Johnson* and went with Redford instead. Eastwood was moved to *Dirty Harry*. This affected the final script for *Jeremiah Johnson* (something about Redford refusing to eat livers) as Redford was imbued with a sense for the "greater good" as opposed to the savage realities of revenge films. The real Jeremiah "liver-eater" Johnson wasn't as interested in "the beautiful and the good" as he was in removing his eternal enemy's skin from its skull. He killed somewhere between 200 to 300 Crow Indians. He scalped them, ate their livers and lived till 90. He was the original "liver king" and spent nowhere near $11k per month on gear.

Milius was not interested in "good men" in the Aristotelian sense. Becoming good would only be accomplished by doing good, which could only be accomplished by beheading evil (preferably in public); there was no alternative. It was good men that let bad men off easy (compare wordcel Tarantino's *Pulp Fiction* diner scene where Jules lets Pumpkin leave alive). It was good men who obeyed, and if Milius's tumults with executives were any indication, obedience was not a behavior he was interested in cultivating, whether in his own life or in the characters which he brought to life on screen.

One such moment takes place between Harry Callahan and the lieutenant he reports to, a pen-pushing mandarin who gloats to Harry:

"I've never pulled my gun, a fact which I'm quite proud of."

"Well, you're a good man, Lieutenant. A good man always knows his limitations"

Dirty Harry was excoriated by filmcel femcels like the *New Yorker*'s Pauline Kael, calling it a "fascist" film, while most on the Right understood that the Harold Francis Callahan was a taller, quieter, vitalist version of Archie Bunker. As his partner says, "Harry doesn't play any favorites! Harry hates everybody: Limeys, Micks, Hebes, Fat Dagos, Niggers, Honkies, Chinks, you name it."

Harry Callaghan was based upon a Long Beach detective who told Milius, "When I'm put on the case, the verdict is in." This detective was reported to have numerous notches on his own gunbelt. According to Milius "He was more out of *LA Confidential* than *Dirty Harry*, but he was an interesting guy becuase he was in his part time a dog trainer, and he was very gentle in training dogs."

While the literati looked for any reason to trivialize and/or demonize white, middle class anxiety, Milius delivered a cinematic gladiator. Harry was the personification of the "Silent Majority": a white allotrope made up of Scot-Irish heritage Americans and more recently arrived white, hyphenated Americans, all of whom needed a champion to wade into the "dirty" miasma of 1970's lawlessness. Against a backdrop of violent crime (rape doubled and homicide grew by 76% from 1960 to 1970) this blue-eyed, brooding Achilles fights when he wants to and with methods he deems worthy despite the incessant bellowing of whatever Agamemnon is assigned to keep him under heel. Milius's on-screen worlds called for men like Harry; men who were beyond convention, beyond societal norms.

There is no better illustration of this than Milius's retreatment of Joseph Conrad's *Heart of Darkness* in his screenplay for *Apocalypse Now*. Partnering with the auteur talent, Francis Ford Coppolla, Milius re-created Conrad's Kurtz through Brando's portrayal of a man who stared into the abyss and become the monster, a menace to the proper order of things. Kurtz admired the Viet Cong's barbarity, their will to triumph. What the West saw as capricious Kurtz saw as an ability to constantly change in everything but their commitment. No measure was too murderous if it meant advancing self-determination. While the Left passively panned *Apocalypse Now* (among other reasons, they didn't appreciate the use of Conrad, TS Eliot and Fraser's *Golden Bough* as literary inspiration), they excoriated *Conan the Barbarian*, with one insider commenting to Milius that the "movie would have been very popular at the Nuremburg rallies in 1936."

"Conan is a barbarian and most of his conflict is with evils that are wrought by civilization. He was a marvelous hero, like Achilles. He sulked and ran away and was force into things and had great rages and great melancholies. He is a character who relies on the animal, and I always believe that the animal instincts in people are the better part of them, and that civilizing instincts are often the worst part of them....contrary to what everyone else says, 'Isn't it better to think and evolve' and all you do when you think and evolve is corrupt yourself... When the going gets tough, the tough get feral."

Conan never becomes an impressive physical specimen without Thulsa Doom's Wheel of Pain. In Milius's case the ratings board assumed the role of Thulsa Doom and their numerous cuts were Milius's own Wheel of Pain. The MPAA gave *Conan* an "X" rating three times, forcing numerous cuts particularly from the raid of the Cimmerian village. One such cut removes Conan's mother hewing down several of Thulsa Doom's men prior to being beheaded in graphic fashion, and a young Conan cutting the throat of a warrior. The novelization of Milius's script gives the reader better insight into Milius's true vision for his cinematic ode to Teutonic savagery.

One scene endured within pop culture's consciousness long after the film had been forgotten by most. The "pit" where Conan cultivated his appetite for blood became inspiration for the UFC's Octagon. When Milius cast Reb Brown in his movie Big Wednesday he didn't realize this would put him in close contact with Rorion Gracie. In their basement dojo, Milius watched them dismantle men twice their size and began introducing members of his tight-knit Hollywood circle into a quasi-Fight Club. Married...with Children actor Ed O'Neill went on to receive a Gracie black belt, calling it the greatest achievement in his life other than his kids, and Milius's own son eventually taught BJJ. Milius's mind envisioned this blood sport as a spectacle of power. He envisioned it playing out in an arena where men could not escape, grappling for supremacy (originally surrounded by a moat of sharks). The early investors of the UFC hired John as their first creative director.

Milius's last, best-known film is arguably one of cinema's best depictions of a mannerbund taking on insurmountable odds. *Red Dawn* depicts a microcosm of society without laws or government which still maintains a semblance honor. While the original story centered on a Lord of the Flies

> **Milius was not interested in "good men" in the Aristotelian sense. Becoming good would only be accomplished by doing good, which could only be accomplished by beheading evil**

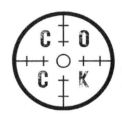

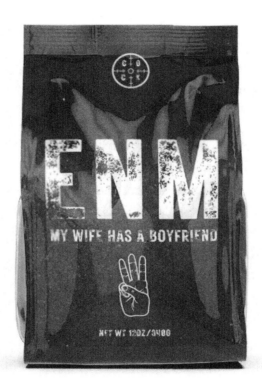

NEW ENM BLEND. MAKE THAT COFFEE FOR THREE.

plotline, with the boys inner depravity becoming the focus, Milius brought an ethos out of the chaos, while still reveling in the idea of lawlessness. He esteemed the concept of a personal Honor Code as more honorable than a society's codification of laws:

"I'm not a reactionary—I'm just a right-wing extremist so far beyond the Christian Identity people... I'm so far beyond that I'm a Maoist. I'm an anarchist. I've always been an anarchist. Any true, real right-winger if he goes far enough hates all form of government, because government should be done to cattle and not human beings."

In *Red Dawn* this honor is primarily underpinned by the martial execution of the "others" yet also rooted in the understanding that true glory, true honor is found in holding out to the last man, plunging sword until steel is broken, the way of the Samurai, the Bushido. Milius found inspiration through the classics and liked the "Song of Roland" in particular. This 11th Century epic tells of Roland at the Battle of Roncevaux Pass in 778. Roland's fighting force of 20,000 is ambushed high in the Pyrenees by the swarthy Basques in retaliation for Charlemagne's destruction of Pamplona. The Frankish commander and his men were cut off and, according to tradition, overrun by 400,000 Muslims. Yet instead of retreating from these insurmountable odds they fought until the last man, allowing Charlemagne to remove the majority of his troops from the treacherous mountains and regroup. Roland and his men established the chivalric model for a medieval knight.

There is no doubt that Milius was inspired to be the last holdout of a bygone era in film history; hardly remembered by most yet hardly caring if he is. Concerning George Lucas's oft-touted leveraging of Homeric heroes, Milius said,

"You know George Lucas talks about it all the time. He doesn't know how to use it at all. He doesn't understand myth at all. As illustrated by *Phantom Menace*. Writers who really understand myth don't use it consciously. There are very few things that are truly mythical. There's a lot of stuff that's famous, but very few things that are the stuff of myth and legend."

While Milius may never achieve the qualities of the former he has undoubtedly distinguished himself with all the qualities and investitures of the latter.

Quotations in this piece are taken from Nat Segaloff, Big Bad John: The John Milius Interviews, *which is out now. Yamnayanage tweets @yamnayanage*

MAN'S WORLD *digest*

WANT TO WRITE FOR MAN'S WORLD?

If you think you've got something to say, email mansworldmagazine@protonmail.com

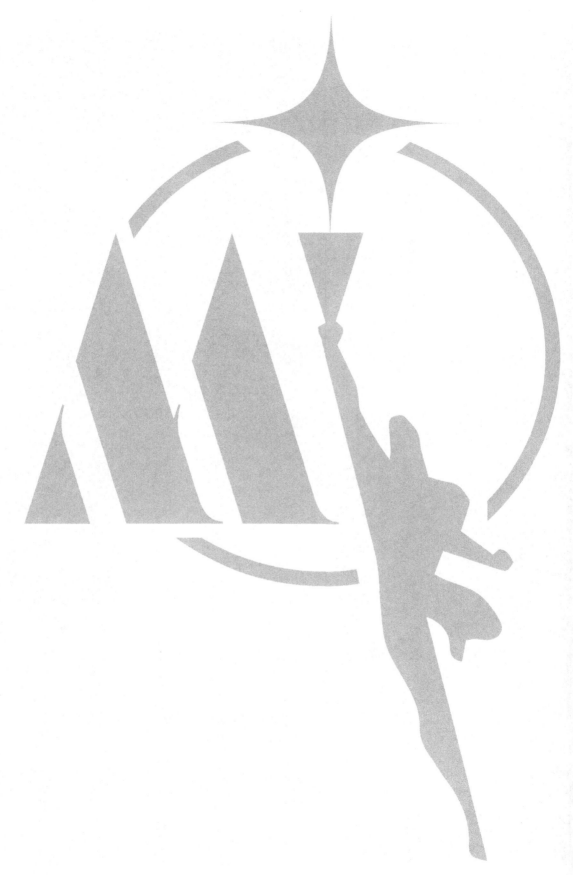

Printed in Great Britain
by Amazon